INTUITIVE
Fasting

The Flexible Four-Week
INTERMITTENT FASTING PLAN
to Recharge Your Metabolism
and Renew Your Health

DR WILL COLE
with Gretchen Lidicker

yellow
kite

First published in the United States in 2021 by Rodale Books,
an imprint of Random House,
a division of Penguin Random House LLC, New York.

First published in Great Britain in 2021 by Yellow Kite
An Imprint of Hodder & Stoughton
An Hachette UK company

1

Jacket and book design by Jennifer K. Beal Davis
Jacket photograph by Julia Gartland

A CIP catalogue record for this title is available from the British Library

Trade Paperback ISBN 978 1 529 37702 6
eBook ISBN 978 1 529 37703 3

Printed and bound in Great Britain by Clays Ltd, Elcograf S.p.A.

Hodder & Stoughton policy is to use papers that are natural, renewable and recyclable products and made from wood grown in sustainable forests. The logging and manufacturing processes are expected to conform to the environmental regulations of the country of origin.

Yellow Kite
Hodder & Stoughton Ltd
Carmelite House
50 Victoria Embankment
London EC4Y 0DZ

www.yellowkitebooks.co.uk

Advance Praise for *Intuitive Fasting*

"In *Intuitive Fasting*, Dr. Will Cole tackles common health issues that stem from our modern eating habits, like chronic inflammation and blood sugar imbalances. His sustainable and customizable fasting plan will help you become metabolically flexible and gives your body a chance to heal itself." **–Frank Lipman, MD, *New York Times* bestselling author of *The New Health Rules***

"My colleague and friend Dr. Will Cole brilliantly shows us how to intermittent fast to gain metabolic flexibility and calm inflammation so we can hear what our body truly needs. Here's to intuitive eating and *Intuitive Fasting*." **–Terry Wahls, MD, IFMCP, bestselling author of *The Wahls Protocol***

"I know Dr. Cole and trust his impressive clinical experience and knowledge, a rare combination. *Intuitive Fasting* provides a flexible and achievable plan for health enhancement that will benefit many." **–Joel Kahn, MD, FACC, author of *The Plant-Based Solution***

"Confused about what to eat? So is your body. But it doesn't have to be! Dr. Will Cole's plan brings back metabolic flexibility and recalibrates our relationships with food. I couldn't recommend it more highly!" **–Daniel Amen, MD, *New York Times* bestselling author of *Change Your Brain, Change Your Life***

"We weren't born eating three squares and snacks, but our bodies are born to feast and fast. This book gives you the tools for doing it seamlessly, easily, and intuitively." **–Jason Wachob, founder and co-CEO of mindbodygreen**

"This excellent guide to eating well will get you in touch with your instinctive eating patterns, helping you become healthier and more mindful about how and when you eat. *Intuitive Fasting* will show you how to finally find metabolic flexibility, so you can intuitively trust your brain and body to function at their full potential!" **–Dr. Caroline Leaf, neuroscientist, mental health expert, bestselling author, and podcast host of *Cleaning Up the Mental Mess***

"Dr. Will Cole is someone I trust for my clients looking for a functional medicine perspective. *Intuitive Fasting* changes the way you view your relationship with food. You'll gain a comprehensive understanding of why intermittent fasting is so effective and how to harness the benefits for yourself. A must-read before diving into the world of fasting." **–Kelly LeVeque, celebrity nutritionist and bestselling author of *Body Love***

"Fasting is a mystery for most. The positive science is clear and credible, and now with Dr. Cole's book you have *the* how-to manual to make this practice more practical. We all need easy, functional solutions with the power to heal the gut, brain, and body—and now you have it, with delicious everyday options!" **–Christopher Gavigan, cofounder of The Honest Company and Prima and bestselling author of *Healthy Child Healthy World***

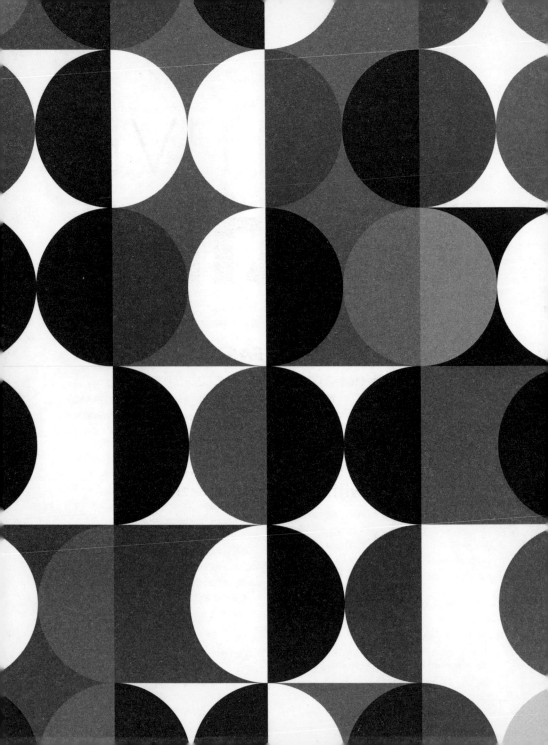

Amber, Solomon, and Shiloh:
Your ineffable love are the embers
behind these pages and my life.
With every breath, I am yours.

Contents

PART THREE: INTUITIVE FASTING: GETTING STARTED AND BEYOND 103

PART FOUR: INTUITIVE FASTING RECIPES AND MEAL PLAN 173

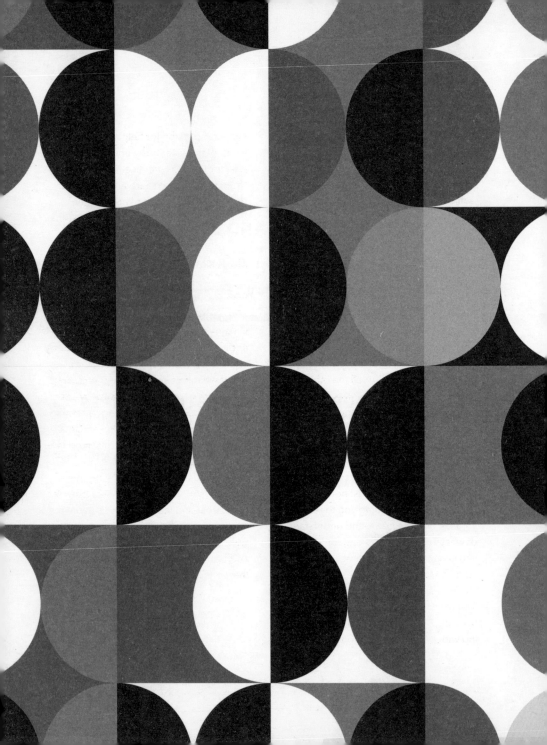

FOREWORD

Of all the different ways of eating I've tried on over the years—from macrobiotic to vegan to I'll-spare-you-the-details cleanses—here is what has worked for me: eating intuitively. When I eat what feels right to me, I feel my best.

That kind of advice, though, is typically delivered with no road map for getting there. As if something that is intuitive doesn't require further discussion, while dogmatic diets get memorialized and memorized.

Will Cole has given me—and you—a road map. *Intuitive Fasting* is Will's clear, four-week program designed to set you up to feel your best for all the other weeks to come. This is not a book of dogma. It will not punish you or restrict you. If there's anything difficult in these pages, it is Will's request that you be willing to listen to yourself, to your own body, to your intuition. While this might seem simple, it is usually not easy, at least not at first. But with Will's voice guiding you to recalibrate yourself and the newfound understanding of what your body is asking for and how you can respond, it becomes doable—and, I'd go so far as to say, exhilarating.

There are healers who share Will's passion for understanding classic research findings. Some share his passion for working with patients one-on-one, while others share his passion for helping the chronically ill or mysteriously unwell patients who arrive at his practice having already "tried it all." Some share his passion for disseminating what he knows to the general public in a way that is accessible. But very few humans share all of these passions. Fewer attempt to sustain them. Fewer find success doing so. And as far as I know, no one does it with the kind of humility and warmth that Will does.

Intuitive Fasting is the best of him: It's what he knows about food and nutrition and the optimal ways to nourish the body and support its healing functions. It's full of what he's learned about reducing inflammation, restoring balance, recharging metabolism, and resetting gut health. Yes, it includes results from research studies, but it also reveals some surprising findings about fasting that Will has discovered from simply listening to his patients. (Another thing I love about Will: He listens—and learns—from his patients.)

It's been a pleasure to witness the Will Cole effect, to watch him help transform and optimize the health of people around the world. I'm excited for you to feel it, too.

—**GWYNETH PALTROW**,
founder and CEO of goop,
November 2020

The Intuitive Fasting Manifesto

A beautiful balance is sewn into the fabric of the universe. Duality is quilted into the cosmos. From the pull of the moon on the tides of the sea, the awakening blooms in springtime after a long winter, to the delicate ebb and flow of your hormones, there is a graceful, dichotomous rhythm infused into nature, of which you are an intrinsic part. Where there is balance, there is order; and when there is a loss of that balance, problems arise.

Our modern world is filled with noisy imbalances of all kinds. From traffic jams in polluted cities to the endless vortex of mind-numbing content online, one thing is for certain—modern life is filled with loud, congested imbalance, dripping in excess.

This global bellowing is not just external, but internal as well. Millions find themselves in a state of proverbial ruckus when it comes to their body and their health. From autoimmune conditions and anxiety to depression and diabetes, heart disease and hormone problems—the consequences of the noise and chaos filling our world are severe. Thankfully, there is a way to get back in touch with the messages your body is trying to send.

Be Still and Know

When was the last time you felt hungry? I'm not talking about the last time you experienced a blood sugar crash, a craving, or the feeling that you "should" eat before a big day at work or a long event. When was the last time you felt truly hungry? When you could feel that your stomach was empty and you could hear it growling and gurgling, letting you know that it's time for a meal?

For many of us in the developed world, it's probably been a while. After all, our lifestyles are designed for convenience and ease—in a way that never leaves us far from a vending machine or a drive-through. Instead of going from full to hungry and back to full again, many of us fluctuate between being sort of hungry, sort of satisfied after eating, and always kind of craving sugar, carbs, and caffeine. Many of us also feel shaky, cranky, or nauseous if we go longer than a few hours without a snack or meal, leaving us with work bags and glove compartments full of granola bars and other healthy—or, more often, not-so-healthy—snacks to help us avoid these uncomfortable symptoms.

Many of us have never paused to ask ourselves questions like: Do I eat because my brain tells me to—or because my body is really, truly hungry? Do I have breakfast because I was told to or because I *actually* wake up hungry? Do I feel more tuned in to my body's natural hunger signals or to the food rules I've been following since I was a kid? Do I feel at peace with—or like a victim of—my daily eating schedule?

What and when we eat has become so ingrained in our culture and lifestyle that many of us have never stopped and asked ourselves if the way we eat is working for us.

The problem is, there's a lot of dieting dogma and food confusion out there. What is ultimately the best food medicine for you may not be for the next person. We are all beautifully and wonderfully unique. Different facets of the same diamond, all reflecting light in our own way. Because of this, I believe using your meals as medicine should be guided by intu-ition. A deep knowing of what your body really needs to fuel and nourish itself.

The good news is that you can get back to a place where you trust your body to send you the right signals. As a result, you'll choose the right foods and lifestyle habits for your particular body. In this book, I'll teach you how to use the transformative tool of intermittent fasting in a fresh and flexible way so you can make the right choices for your health and well-being. Intermittent fasting is a lifestyle practice that involves going specific periods of time without eating, such as leaving a 16-hour window between dinner and breakfast the next day, or only eating every other day. This may seem counterintuitive at the moment. How could intermittent *fasting* get me to a place of intuitive *eating*? Well, I am glad you asked.

For too long, fasting has had a reputation of being overly restrictive and dogmatic. But many of us have been blindly following the "eat three meals a day plus snacks in between" food rules we were taught from day one as we move on autopilot, even if this routine is making us feel unwell.

That also seems restrictive, doesn't it? I think so.

Many of us deal with internal chaos every single hour of every single day. And when your body is out of balance it can be very difficult to discern what your body really does need to build vibrant wellness. It's hard to eat intuitively when you're in a state of imbalance. There's little clarity there. Is it intuition or a craving? Is it intuition or hormone imbalance? Emotional eating is not intuitive eating. Stress eating is not intuitive eating.

As a functional medicine practitioner, my passion is getting to the root cause of chronic health problems, allowing the body to restore its balance and redis-cover calm. I've created the intuitive fasting plan to help you calm down all this noise and start listening to the still, small voice of your intuition that tells you *exactly what to eat and when*. Intuitive fasting is different from other types of fasting in that it's not designed to be difficult or restrictive; it's not about star-vation, it's about self-respect. It's about loving your body enough to perform acts of radiant wellness. Fasting has been used for centuries as a way to strengthen the human body and optimize overall health. Intuitive fasting is about recon-necting us with the way our ancestors did things, because they were really onto something!

Fasting may seem strange at first, but eating mindlessly—and never being fully satisfied—throughout the day is just as strange, if not stranger. When you take a second to step back, it seems a little crazy that we've created these rules around food and meals that we all blindly follow.

In this book, I'm going to ask you to turn on its head everything you think you know about what you eat, when you eat, and how often you eat. Together, we're going to throw out the archaic food rules we've been living by and make our own rules instead. I'm also going to ask you, right now, to drop any misconceptions you may have about intermittent fasting as a whole. I'm going to ask you to enter a new world—a world of dogma-free eating.

Unlike many other intermittent fasting plans, this plan isn't punitive or full of "do this or else" statements—it's simple, actionable, effective, and for everyone. Throughout our journey together, I'll in-troduce you to a lifestyle method that will help you quiet the noise and get in touch with your instinctive eating patterns, not the food rules we've been trained to live by. By doing so, you'll lose weight if you need to, feel more satisfied, increase your energy level, and supercharge your pro-ductivity. In short, you will find your cen-ter. I'll introduce you to fasting through the 4-Week Flexible Fasting Plan, which will get you to a place where you no lon-ger need to obey external expectations about food. The 4-Week Flexible Fasting Plan incorporates multiple unique intermittent fasting protocols to reset your body, recharge your metabolism, renew your cells, and rebalance your hormones. I will also give you a customized food plan to reduce inflammation and support your gut health. I've specifically designed every detail of the 4-Week Flexible Fasting Plan to help you get back in touch with your intuition about food and eating. By the end, you'll feel better than you have in a long time—maybe ever. In four weeks, I'll prove to you that fasting is even more natural than eating three square meals a day, that fluctuating between periods of eating to periods of fasting will feel like the easiest and most natural thing in the world.

I've seen thousands of patients around the world over the years and have helped thousands of people improve their health through my practice and my books. I've seen firsthand how intuitive fasting can elevate a person's health by introducing it to my patients from all over the world; and it has even helped me transform my own health. The program in this book includes recipes, meal plans, and daily eating schedules, so you're never left guessing what you should eat or when. I'll be personally guiding you through the whole process, and you'll never feel like you're swimming upstream.

I believe food and wellness should be fun and magical, and I try to convey that to my patients and through my writing. My first book, *Ketotarian,* was about the alchemy between plant-based and keto diets. My second book, *The Inflammation Spectrum,* was about the transmutation of food confusion into food freedom. This book, *Intuitive Fasting,* is about the awakening of unbounded healing and food peace.

In a world that is out of balance, with this book we are recalibrating, simplifying, and getting out of our heads—*and into our bodies*—when it comes to food.

Ready? Let's ditch the food rules, together.

PART ONE

The New Age of Fasting

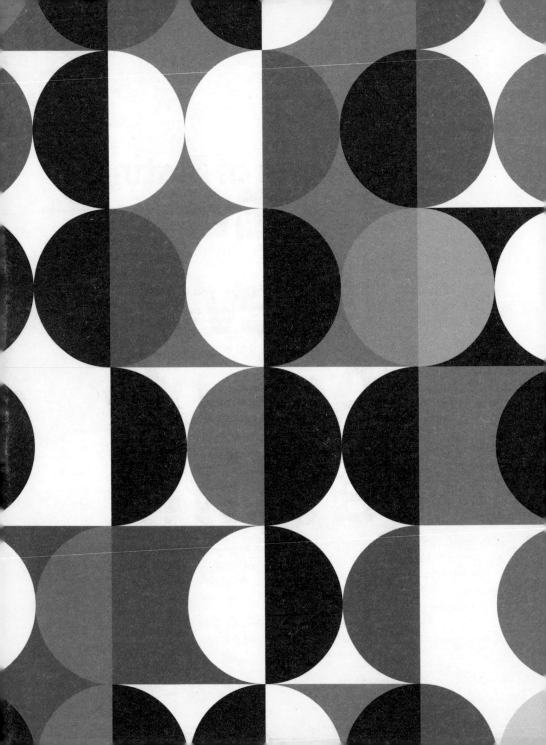

CHAPTER 1

The Origins of Fasting and Food Freedom

If you read the words "intermittent fasting" and a mental image of someone sipping water looking miserable and hungry emerged in your mind, I get it. Intermittent fasting has developed a reputation as extreme and overly restrictive. It's often criticized as a way to prop up a damaging diet culture that is obsessed with weight loss and chasing the "perfect body."

The notion of not eating can trigger preexisting negative thoughts and habits, and, in some cases, following strict dietary rules or fasting can be self-punishment disguised as a wellness practice. It's easy to assume that fasting is just another form of restrictive dieting.

But here's the honest truth: Real intermittent fasting isn't about punishment, calorie restriction, or restriction at all. In fact, these things are the antithesis of the concepts presented in *Intuitive Fasting*.

And yet you'll find that many people will still use "chronic calorie restriction" and "intermittent fasting" synonymously.

Let me be clear: chronic calorie restriction and fasting are not the same things.

Here's what makes them different:

- **Chronic calorie restriction:** Reducing your average daily caloric intake below what is normal for a long period of time.

- **Intermittent fasting:** Limiting how often you eat, or not eating at all, during certain times of the day, week, or month.

See the difference? The key to intermittent fasting is *when* you eat—not how much. Intermittent fasting, especially the type of fasting we'll be practicing in this book, actually has nothing to do with counting calories, chronically restricting food, or eating less overall.

So where does this confusion between fasting and chronic calorie restriction come from? Probably from the fact that one of the practical side effects of intermittent fasting is healthy weight loss. Weight loss is something fasting and calorie restriction do have in common—but that doesn't mean they're the same thing. In fact, somewhat ironically, studies have shown that, for weight loss, fasting can be even more effective than chronically lowering your calories. For example, one study published in the reputable journal *Nature* showed that in 28 obese adults, fasting led to greater weight loss and fat loss than calorie restriction.[1]

If this surprises you, you're not alone. Many of us are still operating under the old logic that weight loss is all about "calories in and calories out," when the reality is that weight loss is much more complicated than this overly simplistic equation. Your body is not a calorie calculator, it is a chemistry lab, and intermittent fasting resets the beautiful biochemistry lab otherwise known as your metabolism.

Intermittent fasting causes fundamental shifts in your body's physiology that help your body burn more fat, feel less hungry, and regain energy—shifts that we'll learn about in depth throughout the course of this book. For now, though, let's focus on the fact that intermittent fasting is simply far easier to maintain than calorie restriction (which can leave you constantly cranky, hangry, and dissatisfied). Most diets fail, and they fail for a reason: chronic caloric restriction will slow down your metabolism and put your body into starvation mode, where it tries to hold on to fat.[2] One study compared the effectiveness of intermittent fasting with continuous calorie restriction and found that intermittent fasting is a great alternative for weight loss, particularly for those who find chronic calorie restriction difficult to maintain.[3]

But wait—aren't we supposed to eat more frequent, small meals a day to keep our metabolism going? Isn't that the healthiest way to live and maintain our weight?

At first glance, this idea seems legit— but the truth is, this theory doesn't hold up when put to the test. One randomized trial using two groups of diabetic patients compared the effects on one group of eating five to six small meals a day to the effects on a second group of eating two larger meals.[4] The number of calories the two groups consumed was the same, but the results showed that two larger meals led to greater weight loss, less hepatic fat content, increased oral glucose insulin sensitivity, and more. In other words, it was better for the metabolism, weight loss, and blood sugar balance to stick to the two larger meals. Our bodies are better able to digest and use the food we eat for usable energy when we eat fewer, larger meals a day.

Other review studies have shown that despite the fact that snacking is meant to keep you from overeating—and snacks can help you feel satisfied temporarily—they don't cause you to eat less at your normal meals, which means you end up consuming more food and calories overall.[5] The results of another study on patients who had recently undergone bariatric surgery showed that higher meal frequency was related to diminished weight loss.[6]

The ideas of "portion control" and "eat small meals throughout the day" have been drilled into our brains. But data from the United Kingdom, published in the *American Journal of Public Health,* indicates that this conventional advice only helps 1 in 210 obese men and 1 in 124 obese women lose weight.[7] Those numbers are shockingly and embarrassingly bad: that is a failure rate of 99.5 percent—and the numbers are even more concerning for morbid obesity. Clearly, the strategies we're currently using aren't working. Looking at those numbers, we're forced to rethink what we've been taught about how to successfully lose weight. The truth is, eating all the time, even if it's only a small amount, costs us a lot. Digesting requires a lot of energy, and it can interfere with other important bodily processes. It's

just plain unnatural to snack before bed, wake up and eat, and then constantly be snacking on granola bars and popcorn throughout the day (however relatively healthy these foods may be).

Another common misconception about fasting is that because fasting can cause weight loss, its health benefits must be attributed to weight loss itself. This theory has actually been studied and disproven.

For example, a randomized trial consisting of 100 women—half of whom followed an intermittent fasting regimen and half of whom followed a 25 percent calorie reduction diet—showed that the women in the two groups lost about the same amount of weight after six months, but the women on the fasting diet had a greater increase in insulin sensitivity and a larger reduction in waist circumference, which will undoubtedly make weight management easier in the long term.[8] Other studies, as cited in a large review paper published in the *New England Journal of Medicine,* have specifically shown that specific benefits of intermittent fasting—such as improvement in glucose regulation, blood pressure, and heart rate, and in the efficacy of endurance and abdominal fat loss—are separate from its effect on weight.[9] As the authors of the paper explain, human and animal studies have shown that the benefits of fasting are not simply the result of fasting-induced weight loss. Instead, they say intermittent fasting awakens powerful healing mechanisms that were lying dormant inside the body. Fasting enhances health and leads to weight loss in ways that are unrelated to a calorie deficit. Instead, fasting triggers shifts in metabolic and hormonal pathways that bring balance back to the body and allow it to maintain a healthy weight more easily, naturally. In short, you can get healthy so that you can lose weight, instead of trying to lose weight to get healthy.

See? I told you I was going to ask you to take everything you knew about fasting and eating and throw it out the window.

The Physician Within: The History of Fasting

Fasting has been pulled into the weight loss world as the newest big wellness trend, which has led to public misconceptions about fasting being just another fad.

But the truth is, fasting isn't new at all.

Name any major religion or spiritual philosophy, and, chances are, it incorporates fasting in some way. In a religious context, going periods of time without food is often a way to gain clarity, show sacrifice, and help one become more responsive to higher powers. In Judaism, Yom Kippur is a day of complete fasting (including not drinking water!) and is considered the holiest day of the year. In Islam, Ramadan is a 28- to 30-day fast, during which food and drinks are not permitted during daylight hours. In Christianity, Lent, the 40 days leading up to Easter, and Advent, the time leading up to Christmas, both started as times of fasting, introspection, and prayer.

In Native American tribes, fasting was practiced before and during a vision quest; the Pueblo people fasted before major ceremonies performed during the change of seasons; shamans believed that fasting allowed them to see their visions more clearly and to control spirits. In ancient Greece, it was thought that eating food increased the risk that demonic forces could enter your body, so the Greeks fasted often. In India, Jainism has various fasting traditions, including not eating to satiation in daily life. The list could go on ad infinitum.

Humans have also been fasting for medical reasons for centuries, long before we had any peer-reviewed scientific studies to back up its benefits. The first records of fasting for health date all the way back to the fifth century BC. Remember Hippocrates, the father of Western medicine? Well, he recommended that his patients abstain from eating or drinking for periods of time if they had certain illnesses or illnesses that needed time and space to heal on their own.[10] The famous healer Paracelsus, who practiced more than five hundred years ago, also wrote about fasting as a great remedy, referring to it as "the physician within."

As the decades came and went, doctors, scientists, and health professionals continued to be intrigued by the health benefits of fasting. By the mid-twentieth century, science had started to catch up with the curiosity of health professionals. Researchers began observing humans and animals while they fasted, recording how fasting affected their health and wellness. They even experimented on themselves. A physician named F. Penny fasted for thirty days, during which he recorded notes on his physical and metabolic markers. In 1909, his notes were published in the *British Medical Journal*.[11] Fasting was used for convulsive disorders—a group of disorders involving muscles contracting and relaxing rapidly (such as in the case of a seizure)—as early as the 1910s.[12] Fasting as a treatment for obesity was recommended as early as 1915, when two doctors, Folin and Denis, recommended short bouts of fasting as a safe and effective strategy to lose weight.[13]

Since then, scientists have confirmed that fasting-induced ketone bodies can be helpful for seizure disorders.[14] By the end of the twentieth century, different methods and philosophies of fasting had begun to pop up as we learned more about how fasting might impact our health in many ways. Today, fasting is studied as a potential treatment for an almost endless list of diseases and dysfunctions, including diabetes, asthma, chronic pain, metabolic syndrome (a cluster of conditions that increases a person's risk

for heart disease), obesity, autoimmune diseases like lupus and multiple sclerosis (MS), and even heart disease and cancer.

The Physiology of Fasting

These days, it seems like there's a new fasting research study being published every single day. Fasting's success in modern medicine is multifaceted, but many of its benefits can be explained by how it aligns humans with the information that's encoded in our genes, connecting us more closely with the way our ancestors lived. That's because while we may have fasted for religious and health reasons throughout history, we have also fasted out of necessity.

Think about it: before there were refrigerators, packaged foods, and drive-throughs, people naturally went long periods of time without food—and our bodies encoded this into our DNA over millennia. It's important to think about the health benefits of fasting from an ancestral and genetic perspective since we are still mostly working with that same DNA today, despite the fact that our lifestyles have changed drastically, especially in the last 100 years. In fact, researchers estimate that 99 percent of our genetics haven't changed in over 10,000 years.[15]

While our genes have remained relatively the same, our lifestyles have transitioned from hunting and gathering societies to farming cultures, which set off an era of food always being readily available. The water we drink, the air we breathe, the soil our food grows in, the food we eat, and how often we eat it have changed dramatically in a very short period of time when seen in the context of the totality of human existence. This has caused a genetic-epigenetic mismatch of sorts: our genome adapted in a way that allows us to cycle in and out of eating—but we are no longer honoring that adaptation, because *we're eating all the time*.

So, why is this a problem? Well, because fasting is literally encoded in our genes, our bodies have evolved to perform certain functions in times of feast and times of famine. For example, autophagy—which is when your body cleans house and recycles dead and damaged cells and proteins—is triggered during periods of time without food. After about 8 to 10 hours without food, your body also enters something called ketosis, which is known for its beneficial effects on the brain and metabolism. Certain mechanisms are activated only in times of fasting, but because many people consume three meals a day with snacks in between, fasting never occurs and these mechanisms can't be activated:

they lie in perpetual slumber. According to researchers, this evolutionary mismatch is at the heart of what is triggering chronic health problems to an extent never before seen in human history—the same chronic health problems many of us are suffering from on a daily basis. And it doesn't end there, either.

As the authors of a study published in *Trends in Cognitive Sciences* theorize, the continuous availability and consumption of food causes changes in epigenetic molecular DNA and protein that negatively impact cognition and can even be passed on to future generations.[16] In other words, this loss of periods of fasting has stunted our healing mechanisms and sabotaged our own health, and we may be passing this confusion on to our children. This is why reconnecting with the way our ancestors lived—through intuitive fasting—is so important. Our bodies have evolved over generations to naturally go for periods of time without food; we are not honoring those adaptations, and the consequences are severe. In the next chapter, we'll explore in greater detail what this mismatch has done to the health of modern humankind, and how many of us are feeling the consequences without even knowing it.

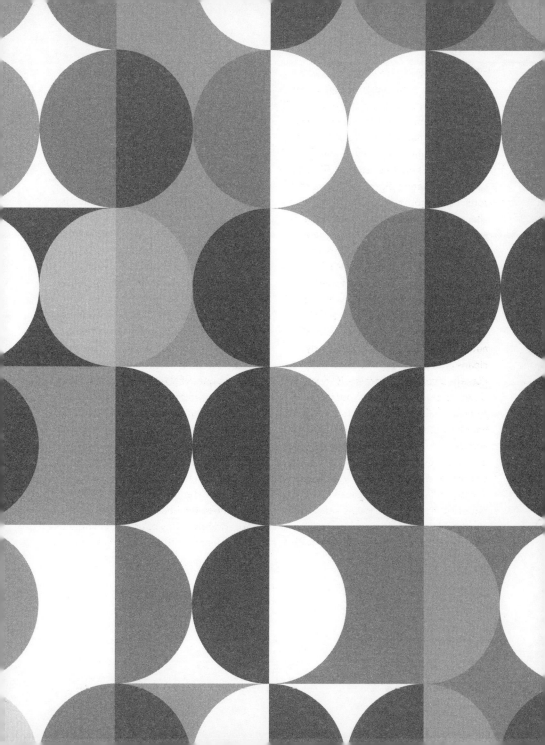

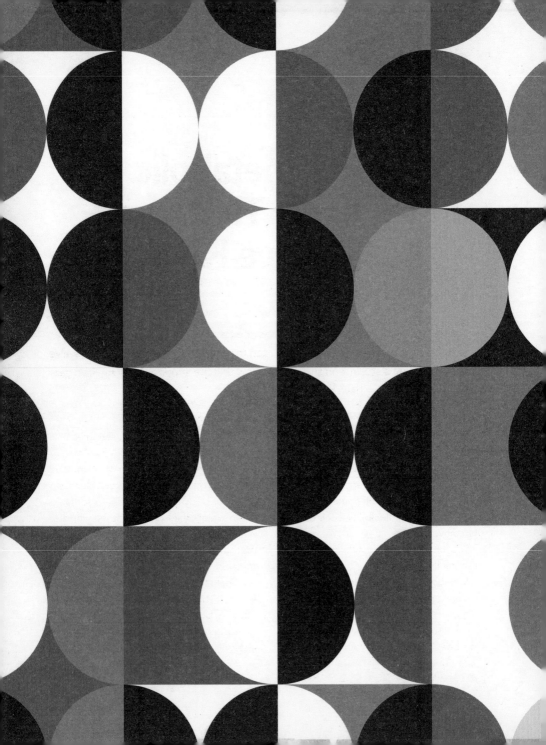

CHAPTER 2

Meet Metabolic Flexibility: The Secret to Intuitive Fasting

As we learned in the previous chapter, over the last few centuries, our bodies have been led astray. They haven't been subjected to periods of time without food; we've been snacking up a storm, and the mechanisms that are supposed to jump into gear during times of fasting have become rusty.

Our bodies have suffered as a result—but so have our intuitions. Thanks to this lack of fasting time, many of us have lost our "metabolic flexibility," a term that will come up throughout the course of this book. Metabolic inflexibility is the death of intuitive eating.

So what does having a flexible metabolism really mean?

Metabolic flexibility is the body's ability to adapt and use whatever fuel is available to it. If you've eaten recently, that fuel is glucose (the sugar that's in your blood). If it's been a while since your last meal (or

all your blood glucose has been used up), that fuel is stored fat. If you've ever entered the "fat-burning" stage of a workout, it means you've used up all your glucose and your body is now burning fat for fuel.

You might think of sugar as the ultimate hit of energy, but, as it turns out, fat is a much more efficient fuel source for your metabolism. Think of it like this: your body is a fire in the fireplace, and the kindling is sugar. This type of fuel provides short, effective bursts of flames to get the fire going, but kindling is quick to burn, doesn't last long, and you have to constantly replenish it to keep the fire burning. The same is true for sugar; you get a temporary energy high and then you crash not long after. If you've ever eaten a bunch of sweets and then crashed hard, feeling like you needed a nap a few hours later, you've experienced this phenomenon firsthand.

In contrast, fat is like a log of firewood. You can put a log in the fire and know that for hours you'll have a slow and steady fire burning. Fat is the same: it provides long-term sustainable, stable energy for your body. Being able to rely on either kindling (sugar) or firewood (fat) to keep your fire going is the definition of metabolic flexibility.

Unfortunately, with our high-sugar, high-carb, constant-snacking culture, it's been a long time since many of us have burned any logs of firewood. In fact, many of us currently rely almost entirely on kindling (glucose) to fuel us and, as a result, our cells have lost their ability to quickly and efficiently switch from using sugar to using fat for fuel. In other words, we've lost our metabolic flexibility and, therefore, our ability to maintain consistent energy levels, brainpower, and appetites.

This can be a difficult concept to grasp, so it's helpful to know where in the body all this is occurring. The answer is the mitochondria. If you're not familiar with this term, the mitochondria are the small energy centers in our cells. They have a few important functions, but above all else, they're responsible for converting oxygen and nutrients into adenosine triphosphate (ATP), which is the main energy currency in the body. When you lose metabolic flexibility, your mitochondria lose their innate ability to efficiently switch between glucose and fat burning to maintain consistent energy levels—a phenomenon that's been coined "mitochondrial indecision," a sort of metabolic purgatory.

The loss of this adaptation can leave us shaky, ravenous, and hangry (have you met her? *hungry* and *angry*'s evil spawn), and—considering the job of the mitochondria is to create cellular energy—extremely fatigued and groggy. We will always be looking for our next hit of sugar, which temporarily pulls us out of our cranky, foggy-brained stupor.

As you can guess, having trillions of cells inside us that behave like mini sugar addicts can make it impossible to connect to our body's intuitive eating patterns. When your body is desperate for sugar because it can't rely on burning fat for fuel, you'll be hungry and craving something sweet, carby (or both!) every few hours no matter how much you eat. Those cravings will be so strong that they'll crowd out your intuition.

Why Metabolic Flexibility Is the Key to Intuitive Eating

As a functional medicine practitioner, I frequently hear from my patients that they struggle with hunger signals and cravings that have gone haywire. "Dr. Cole, why can't I function in the afternoon without a sugar-filled Starbucks latte?" or "Why do I never feel satisfied after a meal?" or "Why do I get unbelievably nauseous and shaky if I don't eat every three hours or so?" are all questions I receive regularly. Unfortunately, feeling like you're never fully satisfied and always looking for the next hit of sugar makes maintaining a healthy weight a challenge, and it can affect wellness, productivity, and quality of life in a major way. It can feel like our whole lives revolve around trying to avoid hunger, blood sugar crashes, and dips in energy—and yes, living that way is exhausting.

As a general rule, if you're craving candy, carbs, and caffeine, that's not your intuition talking. In fact, you should take those yearnings as a big sign that some of the signals in your body have gone haywire and are now sending you the wrong messages.

Let me be clear: if this is you, it's not your fault. As we learned in the previous chapter, we haven't given our bodies adequate rest from eating to get in touch with what they really want and need.

So, what's the key to accessing intuitive eating? The answer is regaining metabolic flexibility, which we will do by reintroducing our bodies to times of fasting. Reestablishing metabolic flexibility is one of the main goals of the 4-Week Flexible Fasting Plan.

Here's a sneak peek of what the plan will look like:

- **Week 1 = Reset:** In Week 1, I'll introduce you to a basic beginner fasting plan that helps you reset your body so you begin to rely on fat for fuel and establish a foundation for metabolic flexibility.

- **Week 2 = Recharge:** In Week 2, you'll be doing moderate fasts with a focus on recharging your metabolism to start regaining the metabolic flexibility you were born with.

- **Week 3 = Renew:** In Week 3, we'll explore the benefits of deeper fasts, focusing on cellular renewal and repair, activating stem cells in order to target chronic inflammation and support longevity.

- **Week 4 = Rebalance:** In Week 4, you'll be cycling in and out of our fat-burning stage and focusing on balancing hormones so that you can maintain metabolic flexibility in the long term.

Let me warn you: At first, fasting might not feel intuitive at all; you'll be fending off cravings and hunger and fatigue. Plus, it will require you to uproot your habits, which can be more difficult than you think.

But once you achieve metabolic flexibility by sticking to the fasting plan and eating the right foods, fasting will become effortless and intuitive. You'll be able to trust your body to function at optimal capacity—which means no weakness, nausea, or crankiness—whether you've eaten 6 minutes ago, 6 hours ago, or 16 hours ago.

That seems pretty great, doesn't it?

It is. But the benefits of the plan don't end with metabolic flexibility, either. In fact, the 4-Week Flexible Fasting Plan is accompanied by a fasting-enhancing high-fat, low-carb, clean nutrition plan that helps you tackle other common health imbalances that are a direct result of our modern habits of snacking and eating a high-sugar, high-carb diet.

These health imbalances aren't necessarily full-blown, diagnosable diseases like diabetes or metabolic syndrome, either. They may be so subtle that your conventional doctor isn't able to spot them. In fact, this chapter may even be the first time you've heard of some of these imbalances at all. But while they may be subtle, they're still playing a role in your inability to be metabolically flexible and your inability to access your intuition about food.

Metabolic inflexibility breeds imbalanced inflammation in the body. *Inflammation* can be a nebulous term, so what is it exactly? It's an essential manifestation of your immune system. Just like advancements in industry or the internet, inflammation is not inherently bad. It is merely subject to the Goldilocks principle: not too much, not too little, but just right, when we need it. When balanced, your body's inflammatory response will save your life. Injuries and infections are healed with the power of balanced inflammation. Conversely, when your immune system is imbalanced, it is a forest fire burning in perpetuity, affecting every cell of your body. This is chronic inflammation.

Imbalance breeds destruction. Just as the earth's climate is thrown out of balance and is warming, an unbalanced immune system is turning against itself in the form of chronic health problems. A sort of global warming of the body. As above, so below.

The good news is that I've designed the 4-Week Flexible Fasting Plan to correct these imbalances, no matter where you are on the inflammation spectrum. On the following pages, I'll explain just what's going on with the body when it's dealing with these imbalances and how the 4-Week Flexible Fasting Plan will address them so that you can eat and fast intuitively and be your healthiest self.

Blood Sugar Imbalances

Chances are good that you or a close friend, a coworker, or a family member has a blood sugar problem; chances are also good that you're not at all aware there is a problem. According to the Centers for Disease Control, more than a third of U.S. adults have pre-diabetes, and more than half of them don't even know it.

But what is a blood sugar imbalance, really? Basically, when you digest your food, the sugars in the food get broken down and enter your bloodstream. Then, with the help of a hormone called insulin, the glucose in your blood is transported into your cells, where it helps provide them with energy. This is a complicated process, and a lot can go wrong, especially if you're not fasting and are eating too much sugar too often.

If there's too much glucose coming into your body too often—and you never take a break from this process by relying on fat for fuel—your insulin receptors get blocked and glucose can no longer get into the cells. As a result, blood glucose levels rise (that is, you get high blood sugar), which leads to pre-diabetes and eventually diabetes.

So what's to blame for this malfunction in insulin? Mostly, what we eat and how often. It's a pretty simple formula, actually: the more sugar you eat, the more glucose you have coming in. The tricky part is that to your body, "sugar" isn't just white table sugar. In fact, sugar can take the form of any simple carbohydrate, including pasta, bread, cereal, juice, desserts, candy, or even "natural" sweeteners like agave syrup or fruit juice. The more often you eat these foods, the more often your body has to go through the whole process of releasing insulin to usher the sugar into your cells. Your insulin will almost definitely have trouble keeping up with this onslaught of sugar, leaving you with excess sugar in your blood but no way to metabolize it. This is called *insulin resistance,* and it's a step

beyond metabolic inflexibility: not only can you not rely on fat for fuel, your ability to use sugar for fuel is also hindered.

If you're concerned about this issue, here are signs that your blood sugar level isn't quite where it should be:

- You crave sweets or breads and pastries . . . a lot.
- Eating sweets doesn't relieve your sugar cravings and even increases them.
- You become irritable and "hangry" if you miss a meal.
- You find yourself needing caffeine to get through the day.
- You become lightheaded if you miss a meal.
- Eating makes you exhausted and in need of a nap.
- It's difficult for you to lose weight.
- You feel weak, shaky, or jittery pretty frequently.
- You have to pee a lot.
- You get agitated, easily upset, or nervous, out of proportion to the reason for these feelings.
- Your memory is not what it used to be.
- Your vision is blurry.
- Your waist measurement is equal to or larger than your hip measurements.
- You have an atypically low sex drive.
- You're always thirsty.

The bad news is that if you have a blood sugar imbalance, going even 8 hours without food can feel like an impossible feat. The good news is that the 4-Week Flexible Fasting Plan in this book is designed to ease you into fasting and to correct blood sugar imbalances at the same time. By fasting and eating a low-carb, high-fat diet, you're giving your insulin receptors a break from all that sugar. That way, you can banish insulin resistance and get back to being metabolically flexible.

Gut Health Issues

When you fast overnight, your body activates a bunch of beneficial mechanisms. But it's also important to know what it's *not* doing, which is digesting. And while it might seem obvious and unimportant, this act of not digesting can benefit your health in more ways than you can imagine.

Hippocrates, known as the father of modern medicine, is known for saying "All disease begins in the gut." These days, research is catching up with him by connecting gut health to other different health issues. The gut plays a role in almost everything happening in our bodies, including, but certainly not limited to, irritable bowel syndrome (IBS), asthma, autism, weight loss resistance, thyroid disorders, autoimmune conditions, and diabetes. You don't even need classic digestive symptoms like bloating, constipation, diarrhea, or acid reflux to have gut problems that are affecting your overall health—and your metabolic flexibility.

But wait, how is gut health related to

our ability to use fat for fuel? The answer lies in the massive population of microbes—including bacteria, fungi, protozoa, and viruses—that live in your gut. This bustling microbiome metropolis, with its diverse neighborhoods of "gut bugs," works with you to perform many necessary functions that benefit your health and metabolism. In fact, a very hot area of research focuses on the link between your microbiome and your food choices, hunger signals, weight, and blood sugar health.

Studies show that patients who are overweight or struggle with weight loss resistance—a symptom of underlying metabolic issues, like metabolic flexibility—tend to have lower microbiome diversity with lower numbers of beneficial microbes and higher numbers of harmful bacteria and fungi.[1] In one fascinating study, scientists were able to transplant the microbiome of diabetic mice into healthy mice to make them diabetic as well, without changing their diets at all.[2, 3] Amazingly, researchers even hypothesize that the success of gastric bypass surgery is due to changes in cravings caused by massive shifts in gut microbiota, not the decrease in stomach volume.

So what does this mean for you? It means that the composition of your gut greatly influences what you want to eat and when. Microbes that feed off simple sugars can even produce toxins and make us feel cranky and tired if we don't eat enough sugar, which explains why cutting it out of our diets can be so difficult.[4] Microbes can also increase our craving for food that they like by changing our taste buds, influencing opioid and cannabinoid receptors, and producing neurotransmitters such as dopamine and serotonin, which are largely in charge of controlling our moods.[5] Pretty scary, right? There's no need to actually fear the bugs in our gut, but we do need to respect their power over us. At the end of the day they know how to make us happy and they know how to make us miserable—and we are very much at their mercy. Our gut health status influences our blood sugar, our metabolic flexibility, and our food choices and cravings.

If we want to become metabolically flexible, tending to our gut health is non-negotiable. The good news is that the 4-Week Flexible Fasting Plan includes foods that feed our beneficial gut bacteria and keep the sugar-eating bacteria at bay. In addition to the delicious, clean foods in the plan, intermittent fasting has also been shown to aid in balancing the microbiome. You will completely transform your gut microbiome so that it helps you crave the right foods instead of the wrong ones. Hello, intuitive eating!

Leptin Resistance

In order to fully understand metabolic inflexibility, we have to talk about leptin resistance. Leptin is a hormone produced in our fat cells, which are not just inactive tissue but an active part of your hormonal systems. One of leptin's main jobs is to tell our brains to use our bodies' fat stores for energy, which is key to metabolic flexibility. Leptin resistance occurs when the hypothalamic cells in the brain stop recognizing leptin's signals. As a result, the brain doesn't perceive that enough food has come in, and it reads that as starvation.

If leptin resistance happens to you, your brain will turn on all the signals it can to make up for the falsely perceived food deficit. Everything you eat goes straight into fat storage, without being used for energy, making the problem even worse. Your brain is saving up for the coming famine, even though there isn't any famine. This can turn your metabolism upside down and make it almost impossible to quell cravings and eat intuitively.

This hormone resistance pattern is one of the most common hidden drivers of weight gain that I find in patients. And it's nearly impossible to turn this condition around yourself. When you're leptin resistant, you could live in the gym and eat like a rabbit and still have trouble losing weight. Correcting a leptin issue is vital to establishing metabolic flexibility and using fat for fuel. In fact, studies have shown that in order for fat burning to occur during a fast, leptin levels *must* also be low.[6]

So what causes leptin resistance in the first place? You might already be able to guess the answer: chronic inflammation.

Inflammation dulls the brain's leptin receptor sites, and it is this impaired signaling that triggers the problem.[7] The body doesn't perceive the leptin that is already there, so it produces more and more in an attempt to get the message through to the brain. High leptin levels are also associated with fatigue, which makes it hard to exercise, which causes more inflammation.

Talk about a snowball effect, right?

If you suspect you have an issue with leptin resistance, you'll be happy to know that intermittent fasting is a powerful tool for decreasing both inflammation and leptin resistance.

Chronic Stress and Brain-Adrenal Dysfunction

If there's one thing we can all probably agree upon, it's that we're all chronically stressed. And, unfortunately, chronic stress does a number on our minds and bodies. In fact, it's estimated that somewhere between 75 and 90 percent of all doctor's office visits are for stress-related ailments and complaints. Stress is no joke: one study published in the medical journal *Molecular Psychiatry* found that chronic stress can actually cause long-term changes in the structure and function of the brain that can contribute to mental health issues.[8] Research from the Behavioral Science and Policy Association found that workplace stress is as detrimental to

your health as secondhand smoke.[9] Other research has shown an association between chronic stress and increased risk of insomnia and even dementia.[10, 11]

So what, exactly, happens when we're chronically stressed, and how is it connected to metabolic flexibility? In one example, a study published in *Biological Psychiatry* found that chronic stress alone can slow your metabolism and increase cravings enough to make you gain more than 10 pounds every year.[12] You see, chronic stress triggers a chain reaction in your brain's hypothalamus, which then sends a message to your adrenal glands (two small glands that sit on top of your kidneys) to release cortisol and adrenaline, which are two of your stress hormones.

Unfortunately for us, cortisol release also causes our blood sugar to rise, which means it can contribute to insulin resistance and sabotage our metabolic flexibility. Chronic stress has also been connected to chronic inflammation and gut health issues. In fact, a study published in the *Journal of Physiology and Pharmacology* suggests that stress is linked to gastrointestinal conditions like IBS (irritable bowel syndrome), GERD (gastroesophageal reflux disease), and ulcers; and another study concluded that chronic psychological stress can be connected to the body losing its ability to regulate its inflammatory response.[13, 14]

One of the most notorious contributors to inflammation is stress, which works with inflammation in a feedback loop: the more stressed you are, the worse your inflammation; and the worse your inflammation, the more stressed you get.

The importance of stress management when you reestablish metabolic flexibility will come up again and again throughout the course of this book. You can eat all the right foods and fast every night for 16 hours, but if you're under extreme psychological stress on a daily basis, your body isn't going to heal and become more metabolically flexible. You've got to show yourself some love, make yourself a priority, and take time to unwind.

The good news is that you don't have to do it alone. In this book, I will help you break the cycle by managing your stress through techniques like meditation, mindfulness, and deep breathing, which will help support your journey toward metabolic flexibility. Then, you'll be able to reconnect with your intuition—and stress eating, emotional eating, and boredom eating will become a thing of the past.

Chronic Inflammation

When you pull back the veil on all the above issues, chronic inflammation is what they all have in common. In my earlier book *The Inflammation Spectrum,* I explain that while the inflammatory response is a positive thing in theory, when inflammation becomes chronic and sustained—owing to factors like a sedentary lifestyle,

inflammatory foods, chemical exposure, and, yes, a lack of fasting and consuming too much sugar—it can lead to symptoms that range from mild weight gain and fatigue to chronic pain and autoimmune disease. Thus it will come as no surprise that identifying and correcting chronic inflammation is another key piece of the metabolic flexibility puzzle.

If you're wondering whether chronic inflammation is an issue for you, here are some classic signs and symptoms to look out for:

- Autoimmune conditions
- Mysterious skin rashes
- Fatigue or low energy
- Excess mucus production
- Pain or achiness in the body
- Brain fog
- Depression or anxiety
- Digestive issues

So how is inflammation related to metabolic flexibility, exactly? Gut-centric inflammation shapes the way we digest, absorb, and use the food we eat for energy. I mentioned earlier that the microbes in people who are overweight and obese are different from those found in people of a healthy weight. Well, it's thought that these alterations cause changes in the immune system that feed low-grade inflammation and trigger metabolic changes—the same metabolic changes that occur with obesity and diabetes.[15]

Chronic inflammation is also deeply

linked to blood sugar health. In fact, chronic inflammation is one of the things that *causes* insulin resistance. In turn, insulin resistance can lead to more chronic inflammation, leaving you stuck in a vicious cycle in which you always want sugar even when too much sugar is what caused your sugar craving in the first place. In addition, visceral fat—the name given to the particularly unhealthy fat that accumulates in the abdomen—produces inflammatory markers, triggering long-term inflammation and increasing a person's risk for metabolic disorders, such as arteriosclerosis and diabetes.[16, 17]

As you can see, inflammation and your metabolism are connected in almost endless ways. And while that might feel like bad news, it's actually a good thing. Why? Because when you start focusing on foods and lifestyle habits, like fasting, that decrease inflammation, you will naturally heal your blood sugar imbalances, gut health issues, and metabolic disorders along with your inflammation.

This is why the food section of this book is so important. We have conclusive evidence that certain foods, which I call the Core4—dairy, sugar, refined grains, and industrial seed oils like canola oil—increase inflammation, so fasting alone isn't enough. We must cut out those inflammatory foods and focus on eating an anti-inflammatory diet full of healthy fats, vegetables, and fiber in order to reestablish metabolic flexibility.

The Metabolic Flexibility Quiz: How Flexible Is Your Metabolism?

Clearly, there's a lot that can go awry with your health, thanks to this mismatch between the way our bodies were designed to live and where we are today as a society. Everything in your body is brilliantly interconnected; metabolic inflexibility is both the underlying driver of these health issues and a consequence of them. The result is a swirling mass of underlying health imbalances that cause you to feel awful on a daily basis. The good news is that by reestablishing metabolic flexibility you are putting a pin in that vicious cycle, turning it into a positive feedback loop instead. With the plan in this book, a new cycle will start with increased metabolic flexibility, which decreases inflammation, heals the gut, and balances blood sugar and leptin, the result of which is more metabolic flexibility. See what I did there? Full circle, interconnected, root-cause wellness.

You may already have an idea from reading the previous material just how much metabolic inflexibility is a problem for you, but I always like to establish a baseline so you can tell how much progress you've made through the course of the plan. To let you find your baseline, I designed the following metabolic flexibility questionnaire. For each statement, give yourself 1, 2, or 3 points based on how true the statement is for you:

1 = not true at all
2 = somewhat true
3 = definitely true

1. You find yourself snacking a lot and always have an emergency snack on hand.

2. You have difficulty skipping a meal.

3. You have frequent or constant cravings for sugar or carbs.

4. You wake up and have breakfast right away, every day.

5. You often find yourself hungry after dinner and eating before bed.

6. The idea of fasting for eighteen hours seems impossible.

7. Your energy levels are inconsistent throughout the day.

8. The 3 p.m. slump hits you hard, and you often wake up groggy.

9. Your brain doesn't work efficiently if you haven't eaten recently; you can't think when you're hungry.

10. You know you lean on caffeine and sugar for energy more than you should.

11. You plan your workouts around your meals and have to time it perfectly so you're not too full or too hungry.

12. You tend to feel hangry or shaky if you don't eat every few hours.

13. You can't work out first thing in the morning without eating first.

14. What you're going to eat and when occupies more of your brain space than you think it should.

15. You often feel hungry right after a meal.

16. When you eat sugar, you don't feel satisfied and instead crave more sugar.

17. You experience anxiety if you have to skip or delay a meal.

18. You rely on carbs or sugary drinks for bursts of energy or brainpower.

19. You feel at the mercy of your hunger and food habits; you are not in control.

20. You know that many of your food choices are made from an emotional place.

21. You sometimes find yourself eating even when you're not hungry.

22. You often use food as a stress reliever.

23. Your previous attempts to cut down on sugar have failed.

24. A life without sugar or bread feels scary and depressing.

25. You often experience brain fog or have difficulty concentrating.

Now add up all of your points. If your score was:

Over 40 Points: Not So Flexible

If this is you, your metabolic flexibility has taken a hit. You likely feel like a victim of your own cravings, hunger signals, mood swings, and energy ups and downs. You probably rely a lot on caffeine or sugar and carbs to regulate your emotions and energy. If this is you, you're not alone. The good news is that there's a ton of room for improvement and you can look forward to the relief that metabolic flexibility will bring to your life. The 4-Week Flexible Fasting Plan is going to bring you measurable, life-changing results! Keep in mind that the first week may be a little bit of a shock for your body, so feel free to repeat Week 1 before moving on to Weeks 2, 3, and 4 if you feel that's what your body needs.

Between 30 and 40 Points: Fairly Flexible

If you scored over 30 points but fewer than 40, you're experiencing some metabolic inflexibility but you're not totally under the control of your hunger and cravings. This is likely because you're already taking some steps to support your metabolism and prevent underlying health imbalances that contribute to metabolic flexibility. That said,

your efforts probably haven't quite done the trick. The good news is that the 4-Week Flexible Fasting Plan is designed to remove all the factors keeping you from true metabolic flexibility by showing you how to approach your metabolic health from a holistic point of view. If this is you, make sure you experiment with Carb-Up days, which may help you take your metabolic flexibility to the next level.

30 Points or Below: Fully Flexible

If you scored 30 points or below, you've already made major strides toward metabolic flexibility and your habits are most likely already metabolically friendly. That said, metabolic flexibility is like a muscle, you have to continuously exercise it or you'll lose it. Plus, if I've learned anything from my years of working with patients around the world, it's that even people who have zero symptoms have some things to optimize or underlying issues they are not aware of. Therefore, if you fall into this group you can think about the 4-Week Flexible Fasting Plan as a tune-up, a preventive, or the way to take your wellness to the next level. Make sure you focus on the Intuitive Fasting Toolbox in chapter 10 and home in on your stress management, sleep, and exercise habits, as well as the fasting schedules.

If your score was high and you have any of the health imbalances mentioned, you're not alone. And while it may feel like you have a long way to go to achieve metabolic flexibility, the truth is, it's not as difficult as you might think, especially now that you have this book.

That's because the 4-Week Flexible Fasting Plan isn't just a fasting plan—it's designed to target and correct metabolic inflexibility, chronic inflammation, gut health issues, chronic stress, and insulin resistance all at once. My plan goes way beyond just fasting. It includes information about what to eat, how and when to exercise, and how to manage stress effectively.

When you complete the plan, you'll be able to trust that your body will be hungry only when it really needs fuel—and that the foods it's craving are the right ones for your body. When you gain metabolic flexibility you finally will be able to quiet the noise of "hangry"-ness, insatiable cravings, sugar-hungry gut bacteria, hormone imbalances, and inflammation to hear what your body truly needs. You'll be able to optimize not just your physical well-being, but your mental well-being.

I know what you're probably thinking. Can intermittent fasting really do all that? What's so great about these mechanisms that jump into gear during times of fasting anyway? In the next chapter I'm going to answer all your "Why fasting?" questions so that you'll have no doubts or hesitations about jumping into the 4-Week Flexible Fasting Plan with passion and gusto.

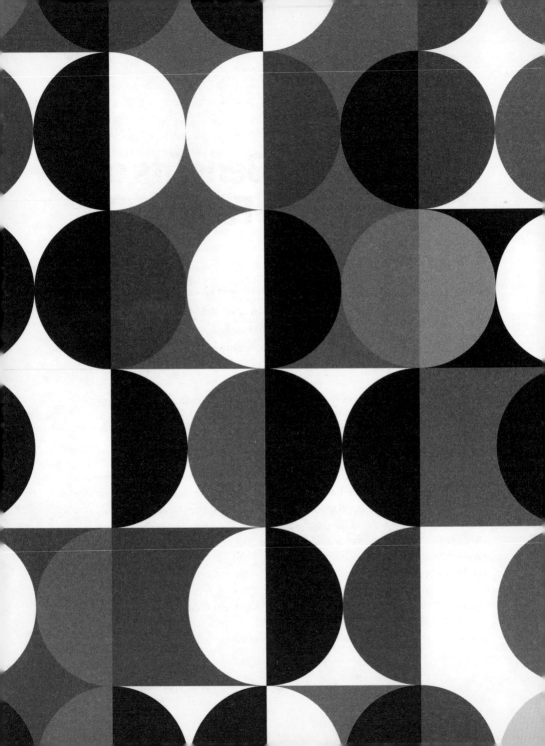

CHAPTER 3

The 5 Key Benefits of Intuitive Fasting

Before we jump into the 4-Week Flexible Fasting Plan, it's important to understand exactly what our goals are—and why, exactly, fasting is so healthy for our bodies. I will explain the benefits of the four different types of intermittent fasting you will experience during the plan, and I will go over some of the core health benefits of intermittent fasting as a whole.

1. Ketosis: The Fourth Macronutrient

One of the main goals of the 4-Week Flexible Fasting Plan is to put your body into different healthy levels of nutritional *ketosis*, a natural metabolic state that kicks into gear when there's not enough glucose (the kindling on the fire that I mentioned earlier) in your blood to use for energy. When there's no sugar to burn for fuel, your body starts using stored sugar in the liver (glycogen) to release usable energy into the bloodstream. Once that runs out, your body starts to use stored fats instead (the sustainably burning firewood on the

fire). This process creates ketones, a type of compound that your liver makes, in the body. When you have ketones circulating, your brain can use them as an alternative fuel source by converting them to energy through a process called beta-oxidation.

So, how do you get into ketosis?

You can get into ketosis a few different ways. The first is by decreasing the carbs and sugars you take into your body so that there is less glucose in your blood to burn and your body turns to stored fat (this way of eating is known as the ketogenic diet).

The second is by limiting eating drastically for an extended period of time (that is, fasting). Unfortunately, with the high-carb, high-sugar standard American diet and a thriving snacking culture, it's been a long time since many of us have been in ketosis at all. The good news is that with intuitive fasting, we'll be strategically using nutrition and fasting to get our bodies into ketosis in a way that minimizes any feelings of restriction and maximizes the benefits of the foods we eat.

The ketogenic diet is a low-carb, high-fat, moderate protein diet that also happens to be the topic of my first book, *Ketotarian*. On a keto diet, you'll lower your carb intake to less than 5 to 15 percent of your total calorie intake for the day (55 grams or fewer of net carbs) while increasing your fat intake to 70 to 90 percent of your total calories. This typically comes out to about 155 to 200 grams of fat a day for someone eating a 2,000-calorie diet. Protein intake on the keto diet is described as moderate, making up about 20 percent of calories (about 100 grams a day).

With the ketogenic diet, you lower blood glucose and force your body to call upon fat to fuel you without having to fast at all. Less blood sugar means less insulin, and as insulin levels fall and your body requires energy, your body releases stored fatty acids from your fat cells into the bloodstream. The ketone bodies made from these fatty acids can be used to fuel your body, just like sugar, but in a more stable and efficient way that allows you to consume far fewer carbohydrates while simultaneously increasing your energy.

In the ketogenic state, ketones in the bloodstream will range between 0.5 and 5 mmol (millimolar concentration), depending on the amount of protein and carbohydrates that you eat. You can measure your ketone bodies with a ketone blood or breath meter or with urine test strips to know how deeply your body is in ketosis, although ketone testing is not required for the plan in this book.

The health benefits of being in ketosis include:

- Weight loss
- Increased energy
- Improved mental clarity
- Better blood pressure
- Improved acne and skin problems
- Lower inflammation throughout the body
- Curbed food cravings
- Reduced (if not eliminated) seizures in people with epilepsy
- Lowered risk of some cancers
- Reversed or improved symptoms of polycystic ovary syndrome (PCOS)
- Improved (if not reversed) type 2 diabetes

So, what makes the keto diet so great? It's the combination of removing sugar, moderating protein, and adding back in healthy fats, thus putting your body into nutritional ketosis, which mimics a lot of the same benefits of fasting.

Most of us already know that sugar is something we should limit. But did you know that it might just be the biggest threat to your health? For many of you, it might even be the one thing keeping you from feeling your best. Americans eat an average of 765 grams of sugar every five days.[1] And today the average American eats and drinks around 130 pounds of added sugar every year, adding up to an astounding 3,550 pounds in a lifetime—that's equal to an industrial-size dumpster full of sugar.

That's a *lot* of sugar. At this point, the dangers of a high-sugar diet are impossible to argue with. Sugar is a known contributing factor to weight gain, heart disease, type 2 diabetes, acne, cancer, depression, anxiety, accelerated aging, fatigue, fatty liver disease, kidney disease, cavities, and cognitive decline—just to name a few.

Even if you decide to reduce the amount of sugar in your diet, accomplishing it is not quite as simple as you think. Much of the sugar we consume is hidden, added where you'd least expect it, or disguised under a different name in the ingredients list of your favorite foods and snacks. In fact, sugar has countless euphemisms, so in order to avoid it, you'll need to know them all and be able to recognize them at a moment's glance. Even foods you'd never expect—like yogurt, ketchup, salad dressings, and pasta sauces—can be high in sugar. In order to reduce sugar, you need to check the nutrition labels of every food you buy and familiarize yourself with the different names it can be disguised under.

Here's the good news: basically all health and nutrition experts agree that sugar is bad for us. In the world of nutrition—which is famous for having many conflicting and dueling opinions and evidence—this is a big deal.

The subject of fat, on the other hand, is much more of a debate among nutrition experts. Fats have been controversial in the past. In the 1980s and '90s, "low-fat" was synonymous with "healthy." In recent years, though, we've discovered that fat is actually essential to our good health—not the disease-promoting, artery-clogging villain we were led to believe. For a long time, there was an endless barrage of misinformation and propaganda against eating fat, with every expert and news channel talking about the connection between fat and heart disease. Now, we know that cholesterol and fat *do not actually cause* heart disease and that lumping fat into one overly reductive category is a big mistake.

The truth is, eating healthy fats like extra-virgin olive oil, olives, avocado oil, avocados, coconut oil, and ghee with vegetables allows your body to better utilize fat-soluble vitamins like vitamins A, D, E, and K_2. Healthy fats are also essential for your cellular health. The foundation on which your body is formed needs these fats to build healthy cell membranes. Don't take this personally, but your brain is your fattest body part, made up of around 60 percent fat (it's okay, mine is too).

Healthy fats also aid in balancing your hormones. Cell communication is key in hormone health, and by eating a diet high in healthy fats you are building up the pathways of communication throughout your body, making it easier for your hormones to convert and get where they need to be. This enables you to become hormonally balanced, which is necessary for your mood, metabolism, and weight. Because our cells, hormones, and brain are all dependent on fats for optimal functioning, we are in effect starving them when we eat a low-fat diet long-term.

That said, a long-term, strict ketogenic diet isn't meant for everyone, which is part of the reason why I wrote my first book. *Ketotarian* is about combining the benefits of a plant-based diet with the benefits of a high-fat ketogenic diet. Some people would rather achieve ketosis through not eating at all for extended periods of time, which brings us to the second way to get into ketosis: intermittent fasting.

The longer you go without food, the more the body naturally burns up the glucose you have stored in your blood. Eventually, you start to run out and the body must call on fat for energy instead, which also produces ketones in the same way as a ketogenic diet. When you've recently eaten, blood levels of ketone bodies are low but begin to rise within 8 to 12 hours after the onset of fasting.[2] Throughout the 4-Week Flexible Fasting Plan, we use both the Ketotarian diet and intermittent fasting to synergistically help your body produce these ketone bodies.

The Benefits of Ketone Bodies

As fasting continues, deeper ketosis develops, you mobilize more stored fat to use as fuel, and ketones end up replacing glucose as the primary energy source for the central nervous system. When we enter ketosis, there are three major types of ketone bodies that are in our bloodstream:

1. Acetoacetate (AcAc) is created first.
2. Beta-hydroxybutyrate (BHB) is created from acetoacetate.
3. Breath acetone (BrAce) is also created from acetoacetate.

These are important to know because individual ketone bodies are responsible for some of the specific health effects of ketosis. For example, in this book, you'll see BHB mentioned a lot. That's because when BHB is produced, it gets transported straight to the brain and enters the mitochondria of brain cells, where it is used to make energy. It's suspected that the production of BHB is responsible for the increased focus and concentration—and the lack of brain fog—that many ketogenic dieters report.

BHB also acts as a signaling molecule in brain cells and can induce the expression of proteins. One such protein, brain-derived neurotrophic factor (BDNF), is known for promoting cellular resilience and synaptic plasticity. This means that BDNF works to support the survival of existing brain cells and encourages the growth of new, healthy ones. Lowered synaptic plasticity has been shown to contribute to a range of brain health, psychiatric, and neurodegenerative disorders, including Alzheimer's disease, autism, schizophrenia, and addiction.[3] BHB also activates the AMPK pathway, which is involved in regulating energy balance and inflammation, and inhibits the NLRP3 inflammasome, an inflammatory protein that activates the inflammatory response and has been connected to various inflammatory and autoimmune diseases.[4] As a result, quite a bit of the research on the health benefits of ketosis is centered around BHB—and each of the three major ketones mentioned has its own healing properties.

Throughout the 4-Week Flexible Fasting Plan, we'll be following a modified ketogenic diet while we ease into fasting. This will help us get into ketosis much more easily (because we won't have a bunch of sugar in our system to burn off before our bodies turn to fat burning). In other words, we'll be accessing ketosis via our food and fasting—more specifically, a type of fasting called time-restricted feeding—at the same time. Talk about double duty! The emerging science on ketones is certainly compelling. It's no wonder they're being touted in the scientific literature as the "fourth macronutrient": proteins, fats, carbohydrates, and ketones. A sort of magical firewood, burning brighter and longer than even the regular firewood of fats.

2. Hormesis: The Secret to Cellular Resilience

The idea that times of starvation are healthy might come as a surprise or feel counterintuitive. I mean, isn't it a good thing that most people have food that is readily available and don't go hungry? Yes and no. Of course, it's a good thing that we've made progress globally when it comes to world hunger and preventing starvation (that's not to say that food insecurity isn't still a very real problem in many places, including the United States). But for a large portion of people living in developed nations where food is readily available—and where processed foods, fast food, and junk foods are often *more affordable* than healthy food—this surplus of convenient food has backfired significantly. Because, as it turns out, intermittent fasting puts the body under a type of stress that can be extremely beneficial.

Wait . . . a different "type" of stress? When I say *stress,* I'm not talking about the psychological chronic stress we all experience while stuck in traffic, looking at our never-ending "to-do" lists, or getting a work call at 11 p.m. The type of stress I'm talking about is *positive stress,* which occurs when you do things like a high-intensity interval training (HIIT) workout, get in an ice bath or sauna, or try to learn a new language or instrument. These things do technically "stress" your body and brain, but they also help you become stronger in the long term. In fact, positive stress has been shown to be so beneficial that there's even a scientific name for it: *hormesis*.

The historical origins of hormesis are quite fascinating. Mithradates VI (135-63 BC), the king of Pontus, a kingdom located in the modern-day eastern Black Sea region of Turkey, had suspected since he was a child that his mother would poison him to death. In an attempt to protect himself from his murderous mother, he would regularly ingest small doses of venom, believing this would defend him against all poisons. Since then, the system of administering nonlethal small doses of venom in an attempt to avert future poisoning has been termed Mithradatism.[5] The sixteenth-century Swiss physician Paracelsus, known as "the father of toxicology," is quoted as saying "All things are poison, and nothing is without poison; the dosage alone makes it so a thing is not a poison," or "the dose makes the poison," an adage reflecting the concept of hormesis. Today's scientific literature further explores this concept.

Something that has a hormetic effect challenges your body, throwing it temporarily off-kilter. In response, your body ramps up growth and repair mechanisms. For instance, in the case of an HIIT workout,

hormesis takes form in your mitochondria—the energy centers of your cells—when they become more efficient. In the long term, HIIT workouts ultimately increase your cells' ability to ramp up energy production. As your body gets better and better at doing this, you develop an adaptive stress response in which you learn to benefit more from sources of healthy stress.

Along with exercise and cold and heat exposure, fasting is one of the major ways to put your body under hormesis. Yes, you are putting your body under a form of temporary stress but, in the long term, you are becoming more adaptable and resilient. This adaptation also occurs on the cellular level: when you fast, your cells enhance their ability to cope under starvation conditions, which makes them healthier and more resilient to disease overall. As long as you don't overdo it and give your body time to recover, you will grow physically stronger in the face of controlled amounts of positive stress, including fasting.

As you can see, a change in perspective is long overdue. Fasting is not just a modern-day wellness trend but a tried-and-true method of safeguarding our health and wellness as humans and honoring the way our genes have evolved over centuries of time on earth.

Intuitive fasting is about moving away from the thinking that fasting is only for those who want to restrict themselves and push their bodies to the limit for fitness or biohacking purposes, and instead seeing fasting as a way to reconnect with our natural way of eating (and resting from eating).

Fasting is a way to put our bodies under balanced amounts of positive stress so they can emerge stronger and more adaptable than ever. We're now rediscovering just how valuable fasting can be—and just how much our health and well-being depend on it.

3. Autophagy: Your Cellular Recycling System

One of the other main benefits of fasting has to do with autophagy, the perfect example of a cellular mechanism that is supported by all types of intermittent fasting. The word *autophagy* was coined by the Nobel Prize–winning biochemist Christian de Duve in 1963, but we've only recently begun to understand just how much this process affects our health on a daily basis. Autophagy (from *auto,* "self" + *phage,* "eat") is a mechanism that jumps into gear during times of fasting in which the body starts to gobble up, recycle, or destroy damaged cells and proteins. At first, this may seem like a bad thing, but the ultimate goal of autophagy is to make room for new, healthy cells to grow and take over. It's been described as "a process of cellular housekeeping," and it's absolutely critical for optimal health.[6]

This process is especially needed when you take into account the onslaught of stressors that our cells are exposed to in modern life. Intermittent fasting has been shown to improve cellular function, increase healing of stem cells, and improve resilience against a wide range of stressors, including metabolic, oxidative, traumatic, and proteotoxic stressors (things like damaged proteins).[7, 8]

Autophagy is important no matter our age, but it's particularly critical as we get older, since aging hinders our ability to clean our old cells and proteins and all this debris can start to build up. Reductions in autophagy have been linked to a range of diseases. The authors of one study wrote that autophagy's main job is to protect us from anything ranging from infections and cancer to neurodegeneration, accelerated aging, and heart disease.[9]

Whenever I talk about fasting to live longer, I'm often met with a lot of raised eyebrows and skeptical looks. But the truth is, until about a decade ago, almost all studies on intermittent fasting focused on aging and longevity—and most of them concluded that fasting can, in fact, improve life span.

Need an example? One of the first studies on fasting reported that the life span of rats increased by as much as 80 percent when they were put on a fasting plan in which they were given food only every other day.[10] In a study on worms, a fasting diet increased life span by 40 percent; in another study on male mice placed on an alternate-day fasting program, researchers observed an increase in longevity.[11]

Okay, but rats and worms are not humans. Well, there is substantial evidence that fasting increases longevity in humans as well. For starters, fasting is known to prevent many age-related diseases, including the top causes of death. There are many theories as to why fasting has such a positive impact on life span. One theory is derived from research on "blue zones," such as the one on the island of Okinawa. The isolated population there typically maintains a regimen of intermittent fasting and has extremely low rates of obesity and diabetes, as well as extreme longevity. As we already know, extended fasting produces ketones; well, ketones also regulate the expression of specific molecules and proteins that play a known role in aging. A few examples of these include NAD+ (nicotinamide adenine dinucleotide, a cofactor central to metabolism) and sirtuins (a type of protein involved in regulating cellular processes, including the aging and death of cells and their resistance to stress).[12] You may have heard of NAD+ because a growing number of nutritional supplements are said to promote NAD+ and, subsequently, a healthier cellular aging process. How, you ask? NAD+ levels decline as you age and, as explained in an article published in *Trends in Cell Biology*, that "may be an Achilles' heel, causing defects in nuclear and mitochondrial functions and resulting in many age-associated pathologies."[13]

It's thought that restoring NAD+ levels,

especially as they decline with age, may ameliorate age-related issues and counteract age-related diseases. NAD+ does this by supporting cellular energy and helping you maintain healthy DNA, but it also does this by activating sirtuins. I'm at risk of diving too deeply into the science of aging, but sirtuins are a class of proteins that occur in all types of living organisms—everything from yeast to bacteria to mammals. In humans, sirtuins play a key role in the body's cellular response to stressors, including oxidative stress and DNA damage. Some studies have pointed to the idea that sirtuins could play a direct role in extending life span. The good news is that NAD+ supplementation isn't the only way to increase the level of sirtuins. In fact, physical activity and dietary changes—including fasting and ketogenic diets—have been shown to increase sirtuins. Even specific compounds, such as curcumin, are being studied for their ability to increase sirtuin levels.[14]

Another pathway that researchers are exploring is mTOR (mammalian target of rapamycin—a central regulator of cell metabolism, growth, proliferation, and survival). Increased mTOR is associated with accelerated aging and age-related disease.[15] The mTOR pathway is especially stimulated by protein consumption. Both fasting and fasting-mimicking diets like the ketogenic diet have been shown to be beneficial at balancing mTOR.[16]

Importantly, intermittent fasting has also been shown to stimulate mitophagy, which is essentially just the autophagy of the mitochondria, and to inhibit pathways that create proteins, pressing Pause on creating new material so that the body can conserve energy and resources while it cleans house. You don't want your cells to always be dividing and replicating, because that has been linked with an increase in oxidative stress. Research has also confirmed that when you are constantly snacking, overeating, or living a sedentary lifestyle, these beneficial pathways are left untapped or even suppressed.[17] This is why giving yourself periods of time without food, regardless of the specific protocol, appears to be overwhelmingly beneficial.

4. Fighting Inflammation: The Sneaky Underlying Illness

With ketosis, autophagy, and hormesis on our side, the potential health benefits of intermittent fasting are practically endless. But there's also one very important benefit of fasting—the ability to help your body fend off chronic inflammation. You'll hear the words "chronic inflammation" throughout the course of this book, and, in the field of integrative and functional medicine, a large majority of the healing process rests on decreasing chronic inflammation and unhealthy inflammatory responses. As we have already learned, inflammation is the underlying commonality in almost every major disease and dysfunction in existence. It makes sense, then, that lowering chronic inflammation would be on the list of intermittent fasting's key benefits.

But how, exactly, does intermittent fasting as a whole work to decrease inflammation? For starters, ketone bodies, autophagy, and hormesis combine to decrease chronic inflammation and bring balance back to the immune system, so fasting decreases inflammation by way of those mechanisms. That said, fasting can also decrease inflammation in a more direct manner. For example, fasting has been shown to reduce the release of pro-inflammatory cells called monocytes, which when circulating at high levels—as a result of the eating habits humans have acquired over the last few centuries—can cause serious tissue damage.[18] Studies have shown that in periods of fasting, these cells go into a type of "sleep mode" and turn off. This means that fasting works essentially as an antidote to the high-sugar, processed food–filled standard American diet.

It's also possible that reductions in inflammation with fasting are due to the anti-inflammatory effects of adiponectin, a protein hormone that's intricately involved in blood sugar control.[19] We learned a little bit about blood sugar imbalances earlier, but about half of Americans have a blood sugar problem, and blood sugar imbalances and inflammation are intricately connected. The improved insulin sensitivity you get with fasting may have direct effects on inflammatory markers, since insulin resistance is so intricately connected to inflammation through cytokines—cells or substances such as interferon, interleukin, and growth factors that are secreted by the immune system to cause inflammation.

We're still not aware of all the mechanisms by which fasting improves inflammatory disease, but we know that in the future, this connection could have real-life practical implications in the treatment and prevention of inflammation-related disease. For example, one study showed that following an alternate-day intermittent fasting plan for a month reduced markers of oxidative stress and inflammation in adults with asthma.[20] This study is a very practical example of how fasting could be used as a therapeutic treatment for inflammatory disorders in the future.

5. Fat Loss: The Body Composition Solution

It's possible that you will lose weight, if you need to, in the first week of this plan. This initial weight loss is largely due to lost water weight and lowered inflammation levels as the body shifts to allow for more metabolic flexibility, but it's also just a natural ripple effect of fasting.

So, while the benefits of fasting go far beyond fat loss, that doesn't mean we should ignore its weight loss benefits completely. After all, maintaining a healthy weight is a crucial part of long-term health.

One study, performed by researchers at the University of Illinois at Chicago,

had 23 obese volunteers follow a time-restricted-eating diet for 12 weeks.[21] The participants ate only between 10 a.m. and 6 p.m., without any restrictions on the type or quantity of food they consumed. The results showed that when compared to matched historical control groups from a previous study, the participants consumed fewer calories overall and lost weight. In fact, the study showed that they ate an average of 350 calories fewer every single day—even though they were not required to count calories or worry about how much they were eating. As one of the researchers on the study said: "There are options for weight loss that do not include calorie counting or eliminating certain foods."

So, how much weight can you expect to lose, exactly? According to a systematic review of 40 existing studies, intermittent fasting is effective for weight loss.[22] The results of all these studies showed that participants who started fasting lost an average of 7 to 11 pounds over a period of 10 weeks. Keep in mind that these studies ranged greatly when it comes to the number of participants—some had as few as 4 and others had more than 300—and the fasting methods (which included all types of intermittent fasting) were followed for anywhere between 2 and 104 weeks, so this number is an average.

Another study showed that simply limiting one's daily eating window to 10 hours for 3 months can lead to significant weight loss.[23] Participants ate only between 8 a.m. and 6 p.m. and lost 3 percent of their body weight, with a 4 percent reduction in abdominal fat. They were not asked to change what they ate, but they did end up naturally consuming 8.6 percent fewer calories.

Fasting's effect on physical appearance goes beyond just weight. Fasting can be beneficial for establishing a healthier body composition and decreasing fat, which are much more important factors to your health than just your body mass index (BMI) or the number on the scale. One study, which put participants on a time-restricted feeding plan, showed increased fat oxidation and weight loss, thanks, in part, to lower ghrelin, our hunger hormone, and less hunger.[24]

Fasting also leads to a drastic increase in human growth hormone, or HGH. HGH is a metabolic protein that is well known for promoting healthy body composition, mainly by increasing muscle gain and aiding fat loss. One study from the Intermountain Medical Center in Utah even showed that during a 24-hour fasting period, HGH levels increased naturally by an average of 1,300 percent for women and by an average of almost 2,000 percent for men.[25]

Unlike chronically restricting your calorie intake, which can lead to the breakdown of both fat and muscle, intermittent fasting has been shown to help you hold on to muscle while you burn fat. For example, one review study showed that when participants on an intermittent

fasting diet lost weight, 90 percent of that weight loss was lost as fat, compared with just 75 percent of weight loss lost as fat on a calorie restriction diet.[26] This means that an intermittent fasting diet plan is more effective at retaining lean muscle.

Fasting might also help target the most dangerous type of fat, called *visceral fat*, which accumulates in the abdominal area around your organs. Visceral fat is particularly damaging because it's hard to lose and puts you at a much higher risk for type 2 diabetes, heart disease, and even certain cancers. Researchers aren't sure exactly why fasting targets belly fat so well, but it probably has something to do with inflammation. What we do know is that visceral fat cells produce more inflammatory markers than regular fat and that, over time, these markers can promote chronic inflammation and increase a person's risk for disease. Intermittent fasting focuses on decreasing chronic inflammation.

Ketosis, hormesis, autophagy, fighting chronic inflammation, and weight loss are the five key benefits of intermittent fasting. You may not be able to see all five of them with your own eyes, but, rest assured, if you're fasting, they are happening behind the scenes, leading to concrete improvements in how your body and brain function. And even more important, they're working hard to lead to measurable improvements in how you feel—in your energy level, cognition, pain level, physical appearance, mood, and even your disease status.

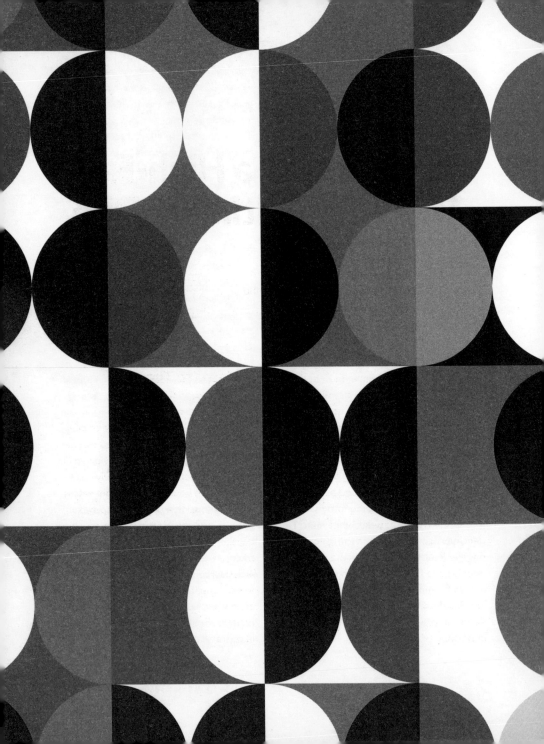

CHAPTER 4

Fasting and a High-Fat Diet—The Ultimate Duo

We often think of "fasting" as a protocol in and of itself; but the truth is, there's more than one way to fast. In fact, there are quite a few different methods out there, each with its own body of research backing it up.

In this book, we'll be following different time-restricted-feeding fasting plans, which encourages total fasting (except for water and liquids like tea) during your "fasting window." We'll also be combining fasting with a high-fat, low-carb diet, which means we'll be getting the benefits of ketosis through fasting and a clean ketogenic-like diet, tapping into many of fasting's health benefits while eating delicious, filling foods. On the following pages, I'll introduce you to time-restricted feeding and the food philosophy we'll be following throughout the 4-Week Flexible Fasting Plan. That way, you'll know exactly what you're doing and—just as important—why.

An Intro to Time-Restricted Feeding

Time-restricted feeding is a type of intermittent fasting that has you focus on when you start and stop eating on any given day. It is typically performed on a daily basis. This can help you avoid late-night eating and help support a healthy sleep-wake cycle. It's also the type of fasting we'll be focusing on throughout the duration of this book. To start with time-restricted feeding, each day, you choose a very specific window of time to eat (your "eating window") and not eat (your "fasting window"). This makes fasting very simple: there's no calorie counting! Really, all you have to worry about is what time of day it is and whether or not you're in your eating window.

Keep in mind that we'll be switching up our exact time-restricted feeding protocol many times throughout the duration of this plan—and that's just scratching the surface of all the different protocols that exist. Throughout the course of this book, I cite research studies that reveal the benefits of restricted feeding, but I also mention studies that have observed the benefits of other types of fasting protocols. Why? Because the 4-Week Flexible Fasting Plan is just what the name says: four weeks long. After it's over, I want you to feel free to experiment with other types of fasting, and I want you to be aware of their benefits. In addition, many types of intermittent fasting seem to encourage similar mechanisms in the body—like autophagy, hormesis, ketosis, and subsequent lowered inflammation—so there is substantial overlap in their benefits. Other fasting plans include:

Modified Fasting Diets

These diets don't require you to fast completely, only to limit your calories to no more than 700 per day on certain days, which can mimic fasting, similar to the ketogenic diet. With a keto diet like Ketotarian, calories do not have to be limited and you can eat until satiety, since its high-fat, moderate-protein, low-carb macronutrient ratio inherently mimics fasting. The modified fasts below are not necessarily focused on food quality, but rather on the temporary lowering of calories to mimic fasting. This will provide you some of the same benefits of fasting.

- **Modified 2-Day Fasting:** With this plan, you will eat a diet full of fresh, whole foods and limited processed and packaged foods for 5 days of the week (which days are up to you), and on the remaining 2 days your calories will be restricted to no more than 700 calories. On restricted days, you can structure your day however works best for you, whether that is smaller meals throughout the day or two moderate-size meals. Again, you'll want to be eating healthy fats, clean meats, and produce. Food-tracking apps like MyFitnessPal or Cronometer allow you to log what you are eating so you can track your calories up to 700.

- **The 5-2 Fasting Plan:** Just like in the modified 2-day plan, you will be eating clean for 5 days of the week. However, the other two days you won't eat anything for 24 hours, and these days must be nonconsecutive. For example, you could fast completely on Sunday and Wednesday.

I chose a time-restricted feeding plan for the 4-Week Flexible Fasting Plan because it's the simplest, least intimidating, and most versatile way to start

LATE-NIGHT SNACKING

Snacking at night after dinner is a force of habit for many of us. We can eat a meal full of healthy fats and protein for dinner, but come 9:30 p.m. many of us are reaching for the cookies, candy, or popcorn. Intermittent fasting is great because, depending on your daily schedule, you can move your eating window around to feel more satiated and avoid eating for the few hours before you go to bed.

Cutting down on late-night eating is one of the major goals of the 4-Week Flexible Fasting Plan. Why? Our bodies have evolved to operate on a daily sleep-wake cycle, which is also known as our circadian rhythm. Our metabolism also works on this daily schedule; it's adapted to eating during the day and sleeping at night, so, naturally, your metabolism slows down in the evening before you fall asleep. If you eat as your metabolism is slowing, it can cause your body to store those calories as fat instead of using them for fuel. Studies on animals show that when they're fed in op-position to their circadian rhythms, it causes them to eat more, gain more weight, and experience more insulin resistance.[1] Knowing this, it's no surprise that late-night eating has been linked to metabolic syndrome and a host of other unfavorable health outcomes in humans as well. Another study showed that eating after 8 p.m. has been associated with higher leptin levels and more weight gain.

Our waistlines and metabolisms aren't the only reasons to avoid late-night eating, either. Deep sleep is when our brains work to consolidate memories, a process that is impaired by eating right before going to sleep, according to a study from the University of California, Los Angeles.[2] I'm telling you all this not to scare you into never having a late-night snack again, but to motivate you to leave at least 2 hours between dinner and sleep. Clearly, eliminating late-night eating is where many of the benefits of the 12-hour fast come from.

fasting—and it's the type of fasting that I do in my everyday life. Time-restricted feeding also helps eliminate late-night snacking, which is a problem for many of us.

It's also easy to combine time-restricted feeding with a high-fat diet that will help supercharge the benefits of your fasting plan, which brings me to . . .

Starting Out with a High (Healthy) Fat Diet

The science-backed plan in this book will lean into fasting by starting slowly with a beginner time-restricted feeding plan, which limits your eating window to 12 hours a day. Typically, time-restricted feeding focuses more on *when* you eat than *what* you eat.

With many other fasting plans, you're not required to change your diet at all. Admittedly, studies do show that to get some of the benefits of fasting, changing your diet is not a requirement. That said, as a functional medicine expert, I'd be remiss if I didn't also give you guidance on what to eat. In my experience in consulting patients around the world, pairing intermittent fasting with a clean, nutrient-dense way of eating will gently lean your body deeper into the fasts and help it rebalance more quickly and efficiently. Eating the foods in this chapter will also make fasting easier, since it will promote better blood sugar balance. If all that

wasn't enough, remember that a clean keto diet actually mimics fasting so that you can leverage many of the benefits of fasting even when you are not actually fasting. This means that if you have trouble keeping to your fasting window at any point throughout the plan, you don't have to stress.

Did you know that you make about two hundred food-related decisions each day? The problem is that most of these food decisions are made on mindless autopilot. As a functional medicine practitioner, I know that the food choices we make every single day can mean the difference between a healthy, energized body and one that feels sluggish and slow. Every single bite of food you eat either helps give your body the ingredients it needs to be its healthiest self, or sabotages it, causing metabolic inflexibility, chronic inflammation, gut health issues, blood sugar imbalance, and other health imbalances. The food we eat throughout the 4-Week Flexible Fasting Plan will supercharge the benefits of fasting, make it easier for you to follow, and support your body's ability to reset, recharge, renew, and rebalance.

So what foods will we be eating? We'll be following a high-fat, low-carb, moderate-protein diet that is not quite a traditional ketogenic diet, but close. You might be wondering why we aren't just following a standard strict ketogenic diet. Knowing the benefits of fats and ketones and the dangers of sugar, the ketogenic diet sounds like the perfect solution—and the keto diet has no doubt taken the wellness world by storm. The ketogenic diet promises to shift your metabolism into a fat-burning powerhouse, allowing you to lose stubborn weight that you may have been holding on to for years. It promises not only weight loss, but also a way to improve your brain function and decrease chronic inflammation, the root factor in just about every chronic health problem we face today. Not to mention, aren't sugar and refined carbs what's sabotaging our metabolic flexibility in the first place?

The problem is that the average ketogenic dieter cuts out sugar and carbs and often replaces them with pounds of processed meats, bacon, beef, cheese, and dairy from factory-farmed animals. These foods are often loaded with antibiotics and hormones, but many keto dieters believe they're fine because they're "low-carb, high-fat." The conventional ketogenic diet also allows you to have sugar-free artificial sweeteners like aspartame, sucralose, and diet drinks, all in the name of being "low-carb." These sweeteners are linked to triggering a whole array of health problems, but as long as they're low-carb and fit the right macronutrient ratio, your average keto dieter will eat them. Because of this hyperfocus on macronutrients over food quality, many people on the ketogenic diet begin to fear and avoid vegetables because of their carbohydrate content. This is a major issue I have with the conventional keto approach.

If the ketogenic diet has so many drawbacks, you might wonder why I don't just suggest a standard strict plant-based diet instead. Typically, these diets are the antithesis of the ketogenic diet: low-fat and high-carb. Advocates of this way of eating tell us that avoiding animal products like meat and dairy not only will reverse and prevent disease and protect our heart health but that it's good for the planet. It is true that opting for more plants instead of meat is said to reduce our carbon footprint and protect against climate change, and I'm a huge supporter of that, but not if we unknowingly sacrifice our own health in the process. This is an issue I see among my vegan and vegetarian patients. Many of them are actually carbatarians, living on bread, pasta, beans, and vegan sweets, all in the name of living green. If they aren't bread heads, they are depending too heavily on soy for their protein, which is typically genetically modified and higher in phytoestrogens. I see many vegans and vegetarians with wrecked digestion and their overall health declining, clinging to their zealous belief that this is the way people should eat and live.

So what's the solution? The Ketotarian Diet. The optimized plan in this book allows us to marry the benefits of a keto diet and the benefits of a mostly plant-based diet—and remove the cons entirely. The Ketotarian lifestyle was born out of my personal journey using food as medicine as well as my clinical experience. The Ketotarian way of eating brings together healthy plant-based fats, clean protein, and the rich, vibrant colors of nutrient-rich vegetables. I'll go over your food list in detail and give you loads of simple, delicious recipes later on in the book, but here's a sneak peek at some Ketotarian staples. First, the foundation of the Ketotarian plate is entirely vegan-keto:

- Avocados/avocado oil
- Olives/extra-virgin olive oil
- Coconut cream, milk, and oil
- Sea vegetables (i.e., nori sheets, dulse flakes)
- Dark leafy vegetables (i.e., spinach, kale)
- Sulfur-rich vegetables, like Brussels sprouts, cabbage, and asparagus
- Nuts and seeds, like macadamias, almonds, walnuts, sesame seeds, flax seeds, and chia seeds
- Low-fructose fruits such as berries

The Ketotarian diet has vegetarian-keto options, so you can add:

- Pasture-raised organic eggs
- Grass-fed ghee (clarified butter)

The Ketotarian diet also has many pescatarian-keto options. This is where you bring in wild-caught fish, like Alaskan salmon, with their beneficial omega-3 fats.

When it comes to macronutrients, you'll be aiming for the following ratios:

- 60 to 75 percent of your calories should come from fat (but it can be more!).
- 15 to 30 percent of your calories should come from protein.
- 5 to 15 percent of your calories should come from carbohydrates. (Most people aim for somewhere between 20 and 55 grams of net carbs daily.)

If you feel great with this macronutrient ratio, there is no reason to eat any more carbs than this. But since we are all different, some people (especially women)—even after they are fat-adapted—feel better eating some more healthy carbs periodically or cyclically.

Clean Carb Cycling

Clean Carb Cycling is a great tool to figure out where your carb sweet spot is and where you feel the best. This is important because eating too many carbs can interfere with your ketone production and blood sugar, but eating too few carbs can also backfire and interfere with your sex hormones, sleep, and weight loss goals. We'll be experimenting with carb cycling in Week 2 and Week 4 of the plan to make sure that doesn't happen. Macronutrient variability is the key to sustainable metabolic flexibility. Here's a preview so you know what to expect: for a few days on Week 2 and Week 4 of the Flexible Fasting Plan, you can increase your net carb intake to 75 to 150 grams per day and reduce your healthy fat intake to compensate for this clean-carb increase. If you've never heard the term "net carbs," here's what that means. We're about to get super sciencey, but basically, total carbohydrates are all carbs found in your food; net carbohydrates, on the other hand, are total carbohydrates minus the fiber and sugar alcohols.

For example:

	Total Carbs (g)	Fiber (g)	Sugar (g)	Net Carbs (g)
1 Avocado	17.1	13.5	1.3	3.6

For whole foods: net carbs = total carbs minus fiber

For packaged foods: count total carbs not net carbs

Carbs from real foods like vegetables and avocados contain both insoluble and soluble fiber. Insoluble fiber such as cellulose and lignin can't be absorbed by the body and has no effect on blood sugar and ketosis. On the other hand, soluble fiber such as galacto-oligosaccharides (GOS) and fructo-oligosaccharides (FOSs) are fermented by the gut microbiome into beneficial end products of bacterial fermentation called short-chain fatty acids (SCFAs): acetate, propionate, and butyrate. The concern in the mainstream ketogenic world is that soluble fiber can increase blood sugar levels, therefore negatively impacting ketosis.

However, studies have shown that soluble fiber can actually lower blood sugar levels. How, you ask? Well, the SCFA propionate is used by the body for intestinal gluconeogenesis (IGN), making glucose in the intestines. Through the IGN pathway, SCFAs actually bring about a net decrease in blood sugar. So, unlike liver (hepatic) gluconeogenesis, IGN seems to have a blood-sugar-balancing effect on the body. If you recall, the beneficial ketone beta-hydroxybutyrate has benefits and structure similar to those of the SCFA butyrate produced from the resistant starch of plant foods.

In addition to all this science stuff, fiber can help with curbing cravings: ketosis + fiber from real food = craving-crushing magic. Win-win. Ketotarianism focuses on nutrient-dense real foods like vegetables, nuts, and seeds, which all contain carbs that are buffered and harnessed by whole-food fiber.

In short: When you are eating non-starchy vegetables, avocados, low-fructose fruits, nuts and seeds on the Ketotarian plan, count net carbs. If you eat processed, boxed foods (even the healthy ones) or any foods other than real whole food, count total carbohydrates.

"Net carbs" are often sometimes referred to as "impact carbs" or "active carbs." Basically, "net carbs" is a more ho-listic way to look at carbohydrate intake.

As you are starting out on your healthy ketogenic path, most people do best with around 20 to 30 grams of net carbs (with a max of 55 grams of net carbs) per day all from non-starchy veggies and whole foods such as nuts and seeds.

For me, Ketotarian goes much deeper than food. Just like intuitive fasting, a Ketotarian way of eating is about food peace. So while you could skip the nutri-tion component of the plan and still get some of the benefits of fasting, knowing what foods make your body thrive and what foods keep you sick and imbalanced is true food peace. And that's what we're learning in this book.

Getting Started

By marrying a nutrient-dense clean keto-genic diet with this progressive form of fasting, you'll be able to get the benefits of ketosis, with all its anti-inflammatory and autophagy-inducing benefits, without having to go too long without food in the first week. Then we'll start stretching and contracting our eating windows to be-come metabolically flexible, sustainably. When we progress to more-advanced fasts, like the ones we take for a spin in Week 3, we'll be limiting our eating win-dow much more drastically. Then, in Week 4, we will allow more wiggle room when it comes to carbohydrate intake. This tailored approach uses both fasting and a clean cyclical ketogenic diet as tools to build resilient metabolic flexibility and, subsequently, radiant wellness.

Before we jump in with both feet, a word on chronic medical conditions. You should absolutely consult your doctor if you have chronic medical conditions such as diabetes, heart disease, or an autoim-mune disorder before you start any fasting plan. That said, having a chronic condition does not mean that you can't fast at all—or

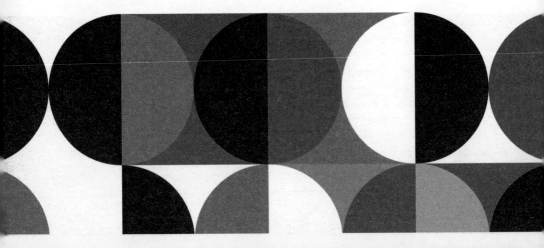

at least find some version of fasting that works for you. In fact, fasting has shown promise for chronic medical conditions ranging from diabetes and Alzheimer's to IBS and obesity (more on that in Part 2 of the book when we talk about the real-life benefits of intuitive fasting). You may simply have to make some adjustments to your fasting program if you have a chronic health issue. For example, you might have to start out slowly or limit your fasts to a certain number of hours.

There is one major exception to this rule, which applies to those with a history of disordered eating, anorexia, bulimia nervosa, or orthorexia (an unhealthy obsession with healthy eating). Research has shown that fasting has the possibility to reignite an overfixation on food. Restricting yourself with regard to food—even if the intention is to improve your health rather than to lose weight—could be a trigger for some people. Disordered eating is the antithesis of *Intuitive Fasting*.

My plan is not disordered eating disguised as a wellness practice. This book is rich with balanced intermittent fasting protocols and filled with nourishing, nutrient-dense foods, but if you've struggled with one of these eating disorders in the past or currently and feel that you'd benefit from this fasting plan, consult your doctor and eating disorder specialist to make sure they give you the go-ahead. Then keep them apprised of any changes to your habits. There is sometimes a fine line between healthy living and obsessive living. If you find yourself hyperfocused on everything that goes on your plate, or thinking that if some fasting is great, more fasting must be better, you've lost sight of the grace that has to be woven into wellness. You can't heal a body you hate. You cannot shame or obsess your way into your wellness.

Now, are you ready to dive into the 4-Week Flexible Fasting Plan?

Let's get to it.

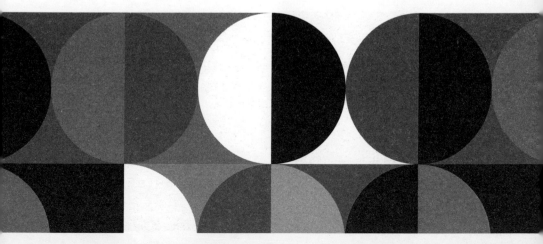

PART TWO

The 4-Week Flexible Fasting Plan

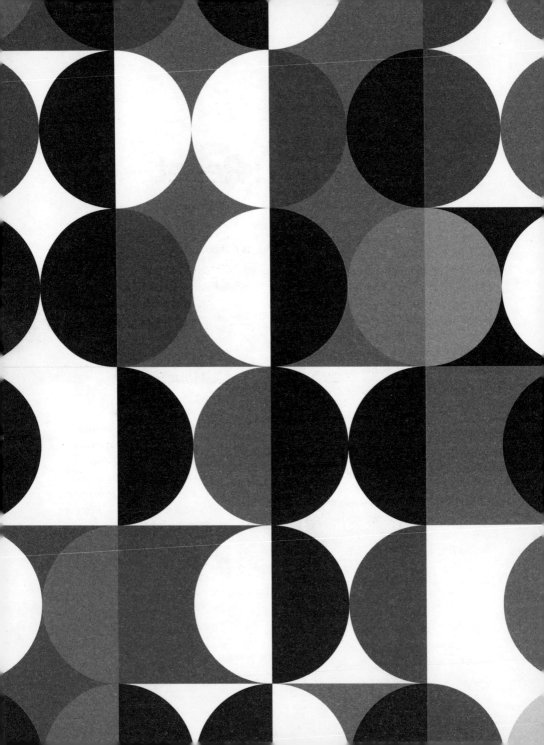

CHAPTER 5

Week 1: Reset

By now I hope I've convinced you that fasting is not about starvation, nor is it just a trendy wellness practice. If you're ready to start fasting to gain metabolic flexibility, then it's time to get started on your 4-Week Flexible Fasting Plan. Over the next four weeks, this plan will take you from relying on constant hits of sugar and carbs for energy to being able to rely on slow-burning fat for sustainable, steady energy levels.

Week 1 is all about resetting your body, creating a foundation that allows for greater metabolic flexibility, and training your body to access fat for fuel, which it may not have done for years. To accomplish this without having to fast for too many hours, we'll be pairing a beginner's fasting method with a low-carb, moderate-protein, high-fat way of eating to enhance the gentle fasting window. This will lean your body into nutritional ketosis through light fasting and a Ketotarian food plan, which means you don't have to jump into the longer fasts right away.

The 12-Hour Body Reset Fast

A light time-restricted feeding window is the best fasting method for starting out because it allows you to get the benefits of fasting without completely upending your daily routine. If I have a patient who is completely new to fasting, the 12-hour fast is almost always where I start. It's perfect for easing your body into fasting and helping you establish basic metabolic flexibility so you can start healing from underlying health imbalances. Once you do that, longer fasts will come more easily and naturally.

It's pretty simple: with this method, you'll easily eat within a 12-hour window and fast for 12 hours every day. At first, 12 hours without food might seem like a lot, but those hours can include the time when you're sleeping. So, in reality, if you're sleeping for 7 to 8 hours, you'll really only be fasting for 3 to 4 hours of the time you're awake each day. You can fast in the morning or at night (or, ideally, a little bit of both!). For example, you could have dinner before 7 p.m. and eat breakfast the next day at 7 a.m. This would give you a 12-hour eating window during the day and a 12-hour fasting window between dinner and breakfast the following morning. You can adapt this in whatever way fits your personal schedule the best, but I recommend fasting for at least 2 hours before you go to sleep. With this beginner plan, you'll be able to access many of the benefits of fasting mostly by avoiding late-night eating—and you won't have to wait too long to eat in the morning if you're accustomed to having breakfast.

I'll go over the full food list and how to easily track macronutrients (healthy fats, clean proteins and carbs) in chapter 9, but for now, here's an example of what your day might look like on the Week 1 Body Reset:

Breakfast: Overnight Lemon-Raspberry Chia Pudding –7:00 a.m.

Lunch: Kale, Brussels Sprout, and Blueberry Salad –12:00 p.m.

Snack: Salted Dark Chocolate–Almond Bark –2:30 p.m.

Dinner: Skewered Tuna with Avocado Salad Salsa –6:00 p.m.

Seems pretty doable, doesn't it? It is. The biggest challenge for many of you this week will be cutting out late-night snacking.

The Real Benefits of the 12-Hour Reset Fast

The two main goals of this week are to eliminate late-night eating and to put your body into ketosis. This allows for the natural production of ketone bodies— which we have already learned has protective and healing benefits for our brains, blood sugar, cardiovascular system, inflammation levels, and metabolism.

This week is where we start setting the foundation for increased metabolic flexibility and begin correcting underlying health imbalances by balancing blood sugar, decreasing inflammation, and giving our guts a 12-hour rest overnight. This week may feel strange, because you're asking your body to go through big metabolic shifts that it's not used to. That said, you may also experience some amazing noticeable benefits from a low-carb diet and a simple time-restricted feeding plan, including less hunger and fewer cravings.

Less Hunger

You might struggle with hunger and cravings the first few days of the fast, but you'll also most likely get to a place where you experience less hunger and feel surprisingly satiated. Why? Because fat provides the body with steady energy and is the most satiating macronutrient, and eliminating carbs will help reduce the blood sugar ups and downs you were likely experiencing before the plan began. Studies have shown that a low-carb diet can help curb hunger.[1]

One of the mechanisms behind this effect of a low-carb diet likely has to do with ghrelin, the body's main hunger hormone. Ghrelin is secreted by your stomach and causes the physical sensations of hunger in your stomach. When ghrelin levels are high, you naturally eat more, store fat, and feel hungry. Thus it's no surprise that we want ghrelin levels to stay low throughout the plan so we can feel less hungry and burn more fat. The good news is that eliminating carbs is also beneficial for balancing ghrelin; conversely, fat is the macronutrient least likely to affect ghrelin levels, and protein is a very satiating nutrient because of its ability to reduce ghrelin levels.[2]

Time-restricted feeding also appears to help with hunger levels. For example, a study by the Obesity Society showed eating dinner in the afternoon improved participants' ability to switch between burning carbs for energy and burning fat for energy—that is, it increased metabolic flexibility.[3] According to the authors, coordinating meals with your circadian rhythms could turn out to be a powerful strategy for reducing appetite and improving overall metabolic health. The results showed that eating dinner in the afternoon and refraining from late-night eating led to more fat burning, less hunger, and lower levels of ghrelin. This is one of the big reasons why I designed this plan to include some sustainable time-restricted feeding protocols instead of other, more-extreme fasting methods. If you are hungry at any point this week, make sure you are eating enough food during your 12-hour eating window. Eat until you are satiated.

Fewer Cravings

If you suffer from frequent sugar or carb cravings, you are not alone. Carbohydrates are extremely addictive; in fact, studies have shown that fast-digesting carbohydrates like bread, soda, and candy can stimulate regions of the brain, called the opioid system, involved in cravings and addiction.[4] And as we already learned, too many high-sugar foods can disrupt our gut bacteria, allowing sugar-eating bacteria to overgrow, which ironically causes us to crave more sugar. The good news is that by following a low-carb diet and leaving a 12-hour fasting window, you are making beneficial shifts in your health that will help you get a handle on cravings.

Just a warning: The first few days of this may be difficult, especially if you tend to eat a lot of carbs and sugar. Studies have shown sugar triggers dopamine release in the same part of the brain that responds to drugs like heroin and cocaine.[5] That means you may actually experience sugar withdrawal symptoms like irritability, fatigue, nausea, and dizziness. For at least the first few days, everything inside you will beg for sugar and carbs. One reason for this is the sugar-eating bacteria in your gut, which begin dying off when they are deprived of sugar. When you start to deprive them of food, there may be a rebound effect in which they cause these uncomfortable symptoms in an effort to get you to feed them.

It's not always an easy feat to cut out sugar, with its addictive qualities and ubiquity in the modern diet, but I will be giving you tools throughout this book so that you can succeed at overcoming sugar addiction. Added sugar also hides behind a myriad of euphemisms, so make sure you read nutrition labels and grow your awareness around how the foods you eat fuel your body. Once you get past the initial sugar detox period, you'll feel better than you have in years. You may find that your cravings subside completely and that you feel totally liberated from sugar. Being in ketosis has been shown in small studies to lead to reduced food and alcohol cravings.[6] By transitioning your metabolism from a sugar-burner to a fat-burner, you're stepping out of the vicious cravings cycle and giving your body what it needs instead of what it wants.

As a result, many people notice a reduction in emotional eating when they start fasting. This is something that I get to see on an hourly basis in consulting with patients around the world; part of the point of fasting is to switch our perspective on food. Instead of feeling like a victim of your cravings, you start to think of food simply as delicious fuel and nourishing meal medicine. You eat to fuel and optimize your body; and the healthier you eat, the better your body functions. Reset week is the initial calming of the noisy imbalance inside of you and gaining metabolic flexibility—the genesis of body intuition.

Body Reset = Gut Reset

The good news is that your gut microbiome starts to respond to fasting and food changes extremely quickly. You might expect it to take weeks or years to change the makeup of your microbiome, but research shows that it can start to happen within a few hours and that significant changes can be observed in just a few days.[7] The 12-hour fast this week is not just a body reset—more specifically, it's a gut reset.

When you are fasting, you are giving your gut a much-needed rest, a gastrointestinal siesta. If you were in the habit of snacking throughout the day and eating late at night before the start of the plan, it's almost definitely been a while since your digestion has had a significant rest. This is a problem because, despite the fact that we often take digestion for granted, it actually requires a ton of energy from our bodies.

Here's what I mean: Digestion requires chewing, saliva production, and swallowing. Then it requires your body to produce stomach acid and your pancreas to release enzymes that help break down the carbs, fat, protein, and starches you consumed into smaller pieces. The pancreas must also release hormones into the blood that help regulate stomach acid, hunger signals, and other digestive processes. Your body produces water, enzymes, bile salts, mucus, and bile that total about two gallons of liquid, which then enters the large intestine. While all this is happening, your gastrointestinal tract has to churn the food and make rhythmic muscular contractions to push the food through your intestines so the food particles, which are now broken down into tiny pieces of fat, protein, and carbs, can be absorbed into your bloodstream and distributed throughout your body.

All this sounds tiring, doesn't it? It is. In fact, it's estimated that we use about 10 percent of our total energy in digestion. And that's on top of all the other bodily functions, like pumping blood, contracting our muscles, filtering our blood and urine, repairing our DNA, and creating new cells that our bodies are already required to do at all times. Many of you didn't realize what you were asking of your body when you had it digesting at all hours of the day and night.

The good news is that leaving a nice long fasting window between dinner and breakfast gives your gut a much-needed rest. The microbiome has its own circadian rhythm and is constantly cycling between different colonies of bacteria throughout the day. When we are sleeping, certain populations of bacteria increase. When we are awake and eat food, others may increase and flourish. This normal microbiome circadian cycle repeats every day but can be hurt when we are eating and snacking incessantly, especially if the food is unhealthy. Time-restricted feeding can help reset the microbiome's natural rhythm. In fact, studies have shown that fasting can reduce the absorption of specific bacterial endotoxins, which have been linked to an increased risk for obesity and insulin resistance.[8] This is particularly relevant if you come into the plan with gut health or digestive issues. In fact, studies have shown that intermittent fasting lowers gut inflammation to help improve inflammatory gut disorders such as Crohn's disease, ulcerative colitis, and irritable bowel syndrome.[9] Another study showed that fasting for 12 hours a day for 1 month significantly improved markers of inflammation, like C-reactive protein and serum interleukin-6.[10] By establishing a 12-hour fasting window, you're also giving your body 12 solid hours a day in which it can take a break from digestion and focus on repairing.

What to Expect During Your 12-Hour Body Reset Fast

If you're completely new to fasting—or have a habit of eating late at night and waking up hungry for breakfast first thing in the morning—you might be nervous about Week 1. I won't sugarcoat it: there may be an uncomfortable adjustment period in the beginning as your body learns to lean on fat for fuel. For most of your life, you most likely haven't thought much about how many hours you spend eating. As a result, your body and brain have come to expect that when you see food, you can eat it. This might make you feel boxed in or a little bit panicked. That's normal and will pass.

You probably also haven't concerned yourself too much with the exact macronutrient ratio of the foods you eat, and you've probably defaulted to a typical American diet that is high in carbohydrates. As a result, every single one of your cells, tissues, and organs has relied on this one quick-energy-producing macronutrient for so long that when you switch from burning dirty sugar for fuel to burning clean fat for fuel, your body can go through a metabolic detox period often referred to as the keto flu. Keto flu can cause symptoms such as:

- Fatigue
- Headache
- Nausea
- Insomnia
- Irritability
- Upset stomach

These symptoms occur because our fat cells often serve as a storage place for toxins like heavy metals and chemical hormone disruptors, which are often found in household products and cosmetics. As we are getting into ketosis this first week, it can trigger the release of stored toxins from your fat cells. And because your gut bacteria feed off what you eat, the change in diet can also shift your gut microbiome; someone with an underlying bacterial imbalance or yeast overgrowth can experience "die-off" symptoms.

Not everyone will experience these symptoms, and if you do, they may not be the same as for the next person. You may never even encounter any of these issues, or you may start off great and then experience mild symptoms after a couple of weeks. If you do experience symptoms of keto flu, I recommend the following:

Drink more water: Make sure you're getting about half of your body weight in ounces of water each day.

Prioritize sleep: You may feel groggy or fatigued this week; make sure you're sleeping at least 7 hours a night. Or, if you're lucky enough to have a flexible schedule, turn your alarm off entirely and take all the extra sleep your body needs.

Don't over-caffeinate: It's tempting to hit the espresso shots of black coffee hard when you're fasting, but I recommend maintaining your normal caffeine intake during the first week of your fast.

Go for a walk: If you're feeling hungry or experiencing cravings, get your body moving.

Don't cut calories: Always eat until you're full during your eating windows. No calorie counting! If you're experiencing symptoms, eat more fat and protein.

If you're experiencing more than minor discomfort from keto flu symptoms, pull back on your fasting window and don't force it. This is where the concept of intuitive fasting comes in. If you find it difficult to make it for 12 hours, start with 9 or 10 hours and slowly inch up to 12 over the course of a week or even 2 weeks.

I mentioned earlier that you may feel "boxed in" by the concept of fasting and that it can even cause anxiety. This is something to watch carefully, especially if you have a hypothalamic-pituitary-adrenal (HPA) axis dysfunction or you're chronically stressed going into the plan. I've found that people with dysfunctions with their circadian rhythms can have a harder time fasting in the beginning, so if this is you, be extra gentle on yourself and make sure you read the stress section in the Intuitive Fasting Toolbox in chapter 10. This Week 1 Reset fast is designed to gently lean you into a fasting and low-carb diet, but if you're not feeling adjusted by the end of the week,

repeat it! There's absolutely no shame in that. Being flexible and intuitive sometimes means leaning in at our own pace.

Week 1 Goals

The goal of Week 1 is to fast for 12 hours every single night for 7 nights in a row. And while 12 hours might not seem like a lot at first, the truth is, the benefits of this kind of fasting plan—especially when amplified with a fasting-mimicking clean, mostly plant-based low-carb diet—can't be underestimated. In fact, if a 12-hour fast every night between dinner and breakfast the next day is all you take away from this book, you'd still be doing your body a world of good.

This week is all about transitioning to fat burning in the gentlest but most efficient way possible. It's important to **follow the plan as closely as possible this week**, especially when it comes to your sugar and carbohydrate intake. Even one small hard candy or a few bites of a muffin can sabotage your progress toward becoming an efficient fat-burner, so this is not the week to be laissez-faire about what you eat. The good news is that if you're able to stick closely to the plan this week, the next 3 weeks will be so much easier. That's because you'll have a solid foundation for metabolic flexibility and you will have reset your gut bacteria and hunger signals. This will all help optimize your body to take on more advanced fasting methods in Week 2.

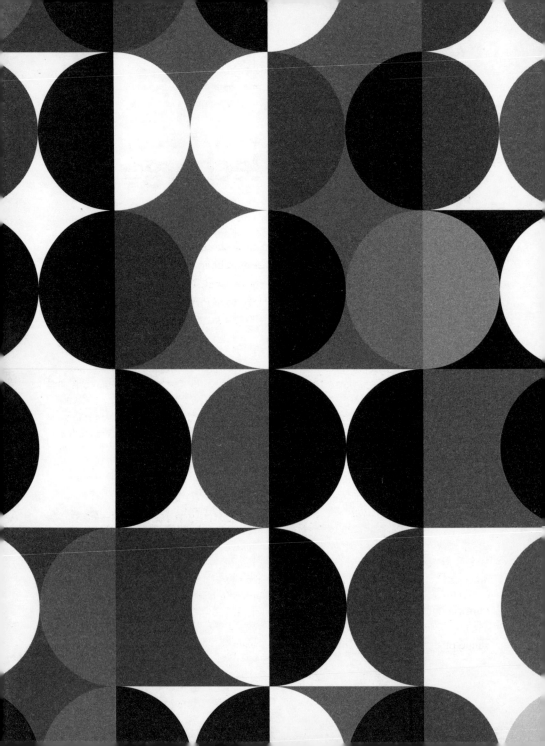

CHAPTER 6

Week 2: Recharge

Welcome to Week 2, my friend. Last week was all about leaning the body gently into ketosis and establishing a firm foundation for metabolic flexibility. This week is all about recharging your metabolism to work for you instead of against you. You'll experience major changes in the way you feel this week—the result of major metabolic improvements that will have lasting changes in the way your body utilizes energy.

We'll accomplish these changes by increasing our fasting window to 14 to 18 hours, thus putting your body deeper into ketosis and giving it a longer period of time to recharge your metabolism and activate the powerful healing mechanisms that occur during times of fasting. This will lead to deeper fasting benefits than you experienced in Week 1, including improved metabolic markers.

We will also be experimenting with Clean-Carb Cycling this week, which means you can increase your carb intake on certain days if you feel your body would benefit from it (we call these Clean Carb-Up days). This is not mandatory—if you feel great on the low-carb Ketotarian eating plan, keep it up—but you have the

option to have more macronutrient flexibility this week if you want it. Week 2 is all about going a little deeper, both in your fasts and in your knowledge of nutrition and what your body really requires to feel its best.

The 14- to 18-Hour Metabolism Recharge Fast

This week we'll be following an intermediate time-restricted feeding plan, which is the same as the beginner plan except that you'll be fasting for 14 to 18 hours instead of 12. I don't give you an exact time frame because this is an *intuitive* fasting plan; I want you to aim for at least 14 hours, and if you're feeling well, you can extend your fast for as long as 18 hours. So, in one example, you would finish dinner at 6 p.m. and refrain from eating your first meal until 8 a.m. (a 14-hour fast) or noon the next day (an 18-hour fast).

This type of plan is what I personally do during the workweek. Since I love the simplicity of waking up in the morning and not having to make breakfast, I like to sip on a few cups of Earl Grey, green, or herbal tea throughout the morning while I am consulting patients online and break my fast at lunchtime. With this plan, you'll be getting a full 14 to 18 hours of fasting, which means your eating window will be carved down to just 6 to 10 hours.

Don't forget, I will go over the full food list in chapter 9, but here is an example of what a day in the life of the Week 2 Metabolism Recharge might look like:

Breakfast: Tea or coffee and plenty of water

Lunch: Kale Caesar Salad with Eggs –12:00 p.m.

Snack: Coconut Lime Smoothie with a side of macadamia nuts –2:30 p.m.

Dinner: Buttery Sea Scallops on Garlic Snow Peas with Jicama and Fresh Mint Salad –5:30 p.m.

What you eat is especially important at your first meal of the day—when you break your fast. As a general rule, this meal needs to contain some healthy fats, like those found in olive oil, avocado, and nuts and seeds. In the example meal plan above, the kale Caesar salad with eggs—full of fiber, clean protein, healthy fats, and leafy greens—is the perfect break-fast meal choice. If you're not inspired by the meal plan just listed (it's okay, I won't take it personally), don't worry, there are plenty of other delicious suggestions and recipes later in the book. For instance, this book includes an entire section on the perfect break-fast meals.

Cyclical Ketotarian: Clean Carb-Up Days

Last week you lowered your carbs—the carbs you did eat came primarily from non-starchy vegetables and low-fructose fruits—which gave your body some time to make the switch from being a sugar-burner to being a fat-burner. This week, we'll be experimenting with the Clean Carb Cycling we learned about in chapter 4. On your optional 1 or 2 Clean Carb-Up days, where you'll be increasing your net carb intake to 75 to 150 grams per day and reducing your healthy fat intake, try adding in more clean-carb options, such as low-fructose fruit, rice, or some starchy vegetables. Keep in mind that a carb-up day is not an excuse to indulge in pastries, pasta, or white bread. Some additional choices include:

- Blueberries (18 grams net carbs per 1 cup)

- Pineapple (20 grams net carbs per 1 cup)
- Baked sweet potato (23 grams net carbs per potato)
- Baked yam (33 grams net carbs per yam)
- White rice (70 grams net carbs per ½ cup cooked rice)

There should be no shame in eating more of these healthy carbs if this is what makes you feel your best. In chapter 8, I'll explain why it is that some people benefit from more carbs and what underlying mechanisms are at play. If you are going to increase your carbs to these levels, I suggest having them around dinnertime to avoid throwing off your metabolism during the day. By having your carbs in the evening, you also can capitalize on their fatiguing effect to help you wind down before bed. Some people also do well when they increase their carbs before or after a heavy workout.

On the other days, continue to eat your normal high-fat, low-carbohydrate diet (fewer than 55 grams net carbs per day) for 5 to 6 days a week. These Clean Carb-Up days are a great option if you are a woman, if you've hit a weight loss plateau, or if you are struggling with some adrenal or thyroid issues. We'll talk more about Clean-Carb Cycling during our Re-balance week (Week 4), but generally I do not suggest increasing carbohydrates to the higher end of these levels this early on for people who tend to have carb sensitivities, such as those with insulin resistance, diabetes, or inflammatory issues or those

who have more than 10 pounds of weight to lose. If you are one of these people, you tend to be more carb sensitive, so giving your body more time in ketosis can aid in gaining metabolic flexibility faster. And to reiterate, *no one needs* to increase their carbohydrates if they feel great. When you increase your carbs, make sure you take note of how your energy levels, brain function, weight, mood, sleep, and digestion respond. On which days do you feel the best?

You don't have to figure out all this yourself. Food-tracking apps make it super simple to calculate net carbs, fats, and protein. And, ultimately, don't obsess. Keep it simple. Once you get the hang of how foods fuel your body, you will grow your intuition and you won't have to use food-tracking apps long-term if you don't want to. Remember: grace and lightness. Use technology to serve and educate you, then drop it and focus on delicious foods. Experiment this week with a Cyclical Keto-tarian approach.

What to Expect During Week 2

As you attempt your daily 14- to 18-hour fasts, you may notice some initial fatigue while you build more metabolic flexibility. Keep in mind that not every day will feel the same. Some days you might feel energized and excited for your fast and then the next day you might feel cranky, tired, and like you want to give up. Some days you might hit 17 hours of fasting and feel like you could keep going, and other days you might only make it to 14. If you're having trouble, experiment with the Clean Carb-Up days and remember that wherever you are—that's okay. Nowhere in this book will I ever ask you to push your body past its limits. Be gentle with yourself. But before you move on to Week 3, you should make sure you have completed at least one 18-hour fast this week; the remaining days should be at least 14-hour fasting days.

This week you may notice some mood or behavioral effects from your new fasting plan. These effects are not common (studies have shown they usually affect less than 15 percent of people), but you may experience irritability, low energy, hunger, or feeling cold.[1] That said, other studies have shown improvements in measurements of mood and concentration, including increases in self-confidence and mood and reductions in tension, anger, and fatigue.[2] You may also notice some weight loss, as well as increased insulin sensitivity and improvements in metabolic functioning. Even those of you who were struggling with weight loss resistance in the past may finally surmount that plateau. The more closely you followed the plan in Week 1, the more likely you are to experience positive benefits—and the less likely you are to experience negative side effects—in Week 2.

Completing an 18-hour fast can be a challenge for some of us; it requires us not to just go the whole evening without food but to delay our first meal well into the next day. Here are some of my best tips for making these longer fasts a little bit easier:

Sip on tea: Organic tea is a great beverage to lean on when you're fasting. It's more interesting to your taste buds than water and even contains compounds called catechins, which have been linked to a decrease in the hunger hormone ghrelin, meaning it helps make fasting a lot easier. I go into the different benefits of teas in depth in chapter 10.[3]

Make sure you're eating enough at mealtimes: I know I sound like a broken record, but you've added an additional 4 hours of fasting each day, so you'll need to make sure you're getting enough food to sustain yourself. During your eating window, make sure you're eating until you feel full.

Focus on healthy fats and proteins: You're eating less often this week, so focusing on fats and proteins is the way to go. These macronutrients take longer for your body to digest and provide you with a much steadier source of energy. This week, make sure you focus on incorporating some kind of healthy fat and clean protein into every meal and even snacks. Nuts and seeds are high-fat and make a great snack to munch on in between your first and last meal. Any sort of clean protein source with vegetables for dinner will finish off your day of eating.

Do some light exercise: Exercise can help you banish cravings and even decrease hunger; plus, it can help you get your mind off food. Just don't overdo it. Some light jogging, yoga, or a walk outside in nature are the perfect choices for Week 2.

Calm your mind: For some people, fasting can trigger feelings of anxiety or stress. You might be worried about getting lightheaded or not completing your fast. This is normal. If you're feeling nervous, try the 4-7-8 breathing from chapter 10 to get your nervous system back on track. You may just notice that it helps decrease your thoughts about food, too.

The benefits of these moderate fasts go deeper than just hunger signals, weight loss, and cravings. This week, fasting is creating lasting changes in your metabolism, including reducing your risk for insulin resistance and diabetes, as well as for heart disease, high cholesterol, and unhealthy blood lipid levels—to name just a few.

The Benefits of the Recharge Fast

Improved Heart Health

Heart disease is the number one cause of death globally, killing more than 600,000 Americans each year (that's 1 out of every 4 deaths). Heart disease costs the United States hundreds of billions of dollars each year—and that number is expected to

continue to rise, thanks to our sedentary modern lifestyles, low-nutrient diets, and high-stress lives.

The good news is that intermittent fasting has proven to be beneficial for heart health, especially when it comes to risk factors such as unhealthy cholesterol markers, high blood pressure, and unhealthy levels of triglycerides. For example, studies have demonstrated that time-restricted feeding shows promise for modulating a variety of metabolic disease risk factors; the same studies showed that fasting also led to higher levels of "good" cholesterol (called high-density lipoprotein, or HDL, cholesterol) and lower levels of inflammatory "bad" cholesterol particles (called small dense low-density lipoprotein cholesterol particles, or sdLDL-c).[4]

Cholesterol is a waxy fat-like substance. Its main jobs in the body are to help build cells and to make hormones and vitamin D. So how exactly does fasting balance cholesterol? According to a study by researchers from the Intermountain Medical Center in Utah, after about 10 to 12 hours of fasting, the body starts scavenging for other sources of energy throughout the body to sustain itself. As a result, the body pulls (bad) cholesterol from the fat cells and uses it as energy. At first, the researchers were surprised to find that on actual fasting days, cholesterol levels went up. But once the 6-week study period was finished, they noticed that cholesterol levels had decreased by about 12 percent.[5] Essentially, fasting mobilized stored cholesterol and then allowed it to be burned off for energy.

Fasting has also been shown to lower triglyceride levels. Triglycerides are a type of fat (lipid) found in the blood. When you eat, your body converts unused glucose into triglycerides, which are then stored in your fat cells. Essentially, triglycerides are stored energy that your body isn't using. If you regularly eat more calories than you burn off—especially if you eat too many refined grains or simple sugars, smoke cigarettes, or drink alcohol—it's likely that your triglyceride levels are high. This puts you at risk for arteriosclerosis, a condition characterized by narrowing of arteries due to the buildup of fatty plaques that may lead to heart attack, stroke, peripheral artery disease, and even fatty liver disease and pancreatitis. When you fast for long enough, your body calls on these stored triglycerides for energy between meals. When this happens, your body breaks down triglycerides into free fatty acids and glycerol, which the body can use for energy, leading to lower triglyceride levels in the blood.[6] In fact, one small study from Liverpool showed that intermittent fasting—in this case, a 2-day-a-week fasting-mimicking diet—reduced triglyceride levels by 40 percent after meals as compared with a conventional calorie-restricted diet.[7]

Pretty exciting, isn't it? It's nice to know that you're getting immediate benefits of fasting, like decreased cravings and weight loss, as well as long-term heart health benefits. I believe that, eventually, fasting will be prescribed as a treatment for preventing and maybe even reversing coronary heart disease and other inflammatory cardiovascular problems.

Fasting, Blood Sugar, and Diabetes

Earlier in the book, we learned that high blood sugar is a huge contributor to metabolic inflexibility as well as to hunger, cravings, fatigue, and other symptoms. But in this section, we're going even further to learn how intermittent fasting could be used as a treatment for pre-diabetes and even full-blown type 2 diabetes.

First, let's go over what diabetes really is. We often hear the word thrown around, but do you know exactly what's happening in the body when diabetes is occurring? Essentially, diabetes is a condition that occurs when your blood glucose (blood sugar) is too high. This happens when your body can't get enough insulin, a hormone that is supposed to transport glucose from the blood into the body's cells, so our cells can use the sugar for energy in the form of adenosine triphosphate (ATP), the body's main energy currency. Insulin is released by the pancreas after we eat foods that contain sugar and carbohydrates.

Unlike type 1 diabetes, an autoimmune condition in which the pancreas doesn't produce insulin, type 2 diabetes occurs when there is insulin resistance in the body, causing the pancreas to produce an excess of insulin. Common lifestyle practices that can lead to insulin resistance include a high-sugar/high-carb diet, lack of exercise, and chronic stress.

When you are insulin resistant, you have chronically high blood sugar and can experience symptoms like chronic fatigue, excessive thirst, increased hunger, and slowed healing. Blood sugar issues are extremely common. The Centers for Disease Control and Prevention (CDC) estimate that about half the U.S. population is either pre-diabetic or diabetic. That's not a typo. Fifty percent of Americans have a major blood sugar problem, and 1 in 4 of these people don't know they have diabetes, which means they're doing unknown damage to their body every single day. About 90 to 95 percent of diabetes cases are type 2 adult-onset diabetes, which means that almost all of them are lifestyle related. Even more worrying, greater numbers of American children and young adults are being diagnosed with type 2 diabetes than ever before.

Clearly, we need maintainable lifestyle interventions that effectively restore blood sugar health. Enter intermittent fasting, which is a fantastic tool for blood sugar control and can easily be implemented. When patients come in with blood sugar problems, I like to recommend intermittent fasting, because of its proven ability to reduce insulin resistance.[8]

In one example of this ability, research-ers from the University of Alabama conducted a small study on a group of obese men with pre-diabetes.[9] They compared the effects of restricting eating to an 8-hour period of the day (7 a.m. to 3 p.m.) versus eating spread out over 12 hours (between 7 a.m. and 7 p.m.). The results showed that while both groups maintained the same weight after 5 weeks, the 8-hour eating-window group had dramatically lower insulin levels and significantly improved insulin sensitivity. In another small study on 16 people, fasting every other day for 22 days was linked to an impressive 57 percent average decrease in fasting insulin levels.[10]

So how does this work? Studies have shown that ketosis reduces the level of insulin in the blood, which could protect against type 2 diabetes.[11] It also looks like fasting improves the way your body metabolizes sugar. When we stop snacking between meals and leave a large fasting window between dinner and breakfast, our insulin levels are allowed to decrease and our fat cells can then release their stored sugar to be used as energy.

Fasting is such an exciting remedy for high blood sugar and insulin resistance that, when combined with dietary changes, it may even be possible for your doctor to lower your medication or to get you off your medication entirely. For example, one study tested intermittent fasting protocols on three different patients who had all been diagnosed with type 2 diabetes.[12] The patients, who had been taking medication for their condition for more than 10 years, were required to eat a low-carb diet in conjunction with three 24-hour fasts per week. By the end of the trial, not only did each patient lose weight, they were all able to completely discontinue their insulin medication.

That fasting protocol is pretty advanced, but studies have also shown that simple time-restricted feeding, much like the one we're following this week, can improve blood sugar levels. One study, published in the scientific journal *Nutrients,* showed that eating only between 8 a.m. and 2 p.m. improved glycemic control by lowering 24-hour glucose levels, reducing blood sugar spikes, and even improving insulin activity.[13]

If you have diabetes, you should speak to your doctor before adopting a fasting plan—particularly the more advanced deeper fasts. In addition, you should know that fasting might be more difficult in the beginning if you have insulin resistance, and it may take longer for you to experience benefits. Why? As we know, fasting leads to a metabolic switch in our bodies when our glycogen stores are depleted and our bodies must call upon fat for fuel. This switch happens many hours after the cessation of eating and is mediated by a receptor protein called peroxisome proliferator-activated receptor alpha (PPAR-α).[14] Interestingly, a blood sugar imbalance can extend the amount of time the body takes to make this switch to burning fuel for energy. So while fasting can certainly be helpful for those with diabetes, it can at first also be more difficult to accomplish.

Fasting, Energy Level, and Mood

Some of the main symptoms of metabolic inflexibility are fatigue and inconsistent energy levels. And, as we have already learned, our energy levels have everything to do with the mitochondria, the energy powerhouses of our cells that work to take in key nutrients, such as glucose, and break them down to turn into ATP. The good news is that by eliminating carbs and increasing fat, fatigue may resolve itself incredibly quickly, since fat has more energy than sugar. In fact, one unit of sugar produces thirty-six ATP molecules, whereas one unit of fat produces forty-eight ATP molecules. Think about that: fat fundamentally provides us with way more energy than sugar. Not to mention, nutritional ketosis has also been shown to increase mitochondria biogenesis, or the making of new mitochondria.[15] Peel back the layers of metabolism, and the mitochondria are what's left underneath. Our mitochondria are what are supposed to allow us to switch between fuel sources. When we are constantly snacking on high-sugar foods, our mitochondria won't make these transitions quite as easily. In fact, according to a paper published in the journal *Cell,* metabolic inflexibility can cause mitochondrial indecision, impaired fuel switching, and energy dysregulation.[16]

In addition, too much inflammation and oxidative stress—both of which are ameliorated by fasting—are thought to be underlying causes of chronic fatigue.[17] Therefore, don't be surprised if you are shocked by how steady and energized you feel this week. You may start jumping out of bed without grogginess or stiffness and make it through the afternoon without a single yawn. In my own life and my patients' lives, this is one of the most practical, real-life benefits of fasting. Less fatigue means more energy to exercise, spend time with friends, or work on projects you're passionate about—the list is endless. With increased energy levels often comes increased mood. As it turns out, fasting may also directly influence mood in a positive way. In fact, studies have shown that fasting can have antidepressant effects, which may be explained by a profound increase in neuronal autophagy (which is just autophagy of the brain cells) and an increase in serotonin, endorphins, and brain-derived neurotrophic factor (BDNF), a few major contributors to mood regulation.[18, 19, 20]

Week 2 Goals

This week our goal is to lean deeper into our fasts, which means we'll be getting deeper into nutritional ketosis, producing more healing ketone bodies and causing major metabolic shifts. Luckily, our work in Week 1 has prepared your body to burn fat and adapt to longer windows without food. This week we want to strike a balance between extending your fasting window as close to 18 hours as you can without pushing your body past its limit and causing unnecessary stress. Focusing on eating plenty of fat, hydrating, and doing some light exercise will help with that.

You can then sit back and allow your body to make major metabolic shifts that will create lasting health benefits, like tackling underlying insulin resistance and cardiometabolic risk factors such as dyslipidemia (an abnormal amount of lipids in the blood). If you're feeling good this week, enjoy it! If you're still feeling a little bit like you have whiplash from this new clean way of eating and fasting, that's also okay. Massive metabolic changes are going on in your body this week. You've likely spent your entire life eating three meals a day plus a few snacks, and now your eating window has been reduced to just 6 to 10 hours. Either way, listen to what your body is telling you. If it wants extra sleep, more water, and a Clean Carb-Up day—honor that need. If it's feeling like a high-intensity interval training (HIIT) workout, an 18-hour fast, and a night out dancing with friends—honor that need! Next week, I'll have you start to connect even more with your body's intuition, which is slowly becoming stronger and stronger by the day as you establish more and more metabolic flexibility.

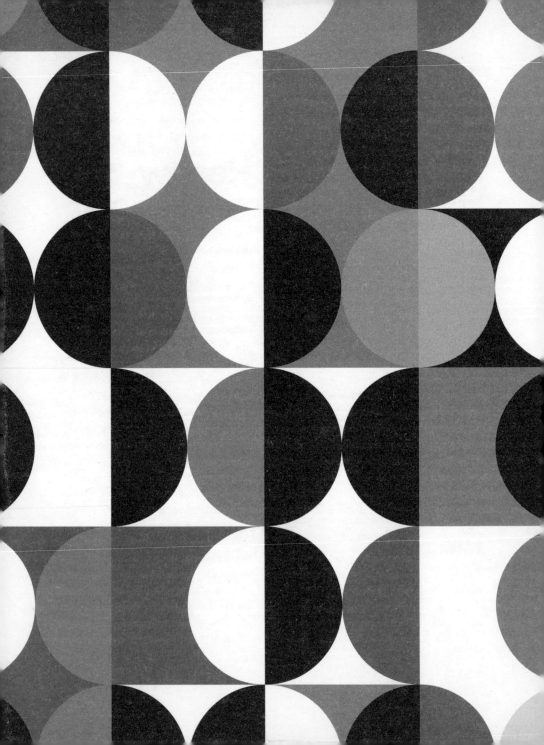

CHAPTER 7

Week 3: Renew

Week 3 is here, you freaking rock star. Over the next 7 days, we'll be doing our longest fasts of all by completing 20- to 22-hour fasts every other day. Our focus this week will be on cellular renewal, and these longer fasts will give mechanisms like autophagy and ketosis plenty of time to really kick into gear and get to work.

As we lean into these longer fasts, we lean into deeper benefits. Studies have shown that longer fasts encourage a shift into nutritional ketosis more than shorter fasting windows.[1] This means in each week of the 4-Week Flexible Fasting Plan, we've been increasing our time in ketosis and deepening our benefits. Short fasts like the ones we did in Week 1 still have a ton of positives, but the fasts we're doing in Week 2 and Week 3 are taking things to a whole new level. This is also the part of the plan where we start stretching and compressing our fasting windows to achieving even greater benefits. Like a proverbial yoga class for your metabolism, you're gaining strength and flexibility. It's also the week when the advantages of fasting get serious—and where we really talk about

disease prevention, longevity, increasing stem cells, and decreasing cellular aging.

Before we jump into the fasting protocol, think back to last week. Did you complete at least one 18-hour fast? If not, you might want to consider repeating Week 2 before you move on to Week 3. This isn't a requirement, but I believe it will better set you up for success in Week 3.

The 20- to 22-Hour Cellular Renewal Fast

Fasting for 20 to 22 hours a day means you'll have time for only one smaller transition meal (what I call a Break-a-Fast meal—more on this in the Intuitive Fasting Toolbox in chapter 10), one main meal, and maybe a snack. Ultimately, your eating window could be any meal at any time, as long as it happens within the 2- to 4-hour eating window of the day.

OMAD, or "one meal a day," is a type of fasting that we will be exploring with an "Almost-OMAD" approach. The reason why I advocate an Almost-OMAD approach by spreading out your eating window to 2 to 4 hours versus the more traditional 24:1 fasting-to-eating OMAD approach is to allow time for you to eat your food in a more gentle, sustainable way for your body. By having a smaller Break-a-Fast meal that is gentle on your gut and then eating your main meal about an hour later, you can maximize the benefits of both your longer fast and your food. Getting all the nutrition you need all at once in a short period of time can be hard on your digestion, and studies have shown it can increase something called the PKR pathway, which can spike meta-flammation, or systemic inflammation.[2] Even my Almost-OMAD approach may seem extreme to you, but after the work you've done increasing your metabolic flexibility in the past two weeks, you might be surprised by how easily you complete these longer fasts. You might also be surprised by the sheer simplicity and convenience of eating only one major meal a day. There is very little meal prep and planning involved this week, which is a far cry from the labor-intensive detoxes and cleanses you may have done in the past.

The only real question you need to answer this week is when to break your fast and how you will fit enough calories and nutrients for the day into one single meal. To do this, you'll have to incorporate how many calories and nutrients you need for your age, weight, and activity level, then make sure your one big meal of the day is full of nutrient-dense real food. Luckily, in the recipe section, there are plenty of meals that contain enough calories and nutrients to fuel you until your next eating window.

Keep in mind that you won't be fasting for this long every day—only every other day, completing 3 to 4 nonconsecutive Almost-OMAD fasts this week. On your non-fasting days, you'll still maintain a 12-hour eating window as you did in Week 1, eating those delicious clean fasting-mimicking Ketotarian foods, with no Clean Carb-Up days this week.

I'll go over your full food list in chapter 9, but here is an example of what a day in the life of your every-other-day 20- to 22-hour Cellular Renewal fast might look like:

Morning: Tea or coffee and plenty of water

Lunchtime: Tea and plenty of water with some added sea salt for electrolytes —12:00 p.m.

Break-a-Fast (smaller, gentle-to-digest meal): Tomato-Arugula Soup —4:00 p.m.

Main Meal: Two poached eggs served over Broccoli-Mushroom Roast with Sesame Seeds, avocado, and toasted cashews –5:00 p.m.

Snack: Strawberry-Spirulina Smoothie –5:30 p.m.

Week 3: What to Expect

This is the week when we lean fully into deeper fasting. You might have felt amazing last week and you might continue to feel amazing this week—despite the fact that you're only eating one and a half meals a day every other day. My patients often report feeling energized and clear-headed when they are at this stage. You can thank 3 weeks of steadily decreasing inflammation levels, increasingly balanced blood sugar, healthier leptin levels, and positive changes in the gut microbiome for this. At this point, your body is seamlessly switching to burning fat for fuel and you're getting deep into ketosis easily.

Here are some tips to make this week easier:

Drink a lot of water: I know I say this every week, but it really is *just that important*. When you're in ketosis, you can lose water weight and that can lead to dehydration and constipation. Make sure you're drinking plenty of water this week—at least eight 8-ounce glasses of pure, filtered water daily—and every week for that matter.

Don't forget your electrolytes: This week, just drinking water won't be enough. Deepening your ketosis like we are this week can also put you at risk for deficiencies in electrolytes like sodium, magnesium, and potassium. The good news is that this can easily be solved by taking some electrolyte supplements or adding a little sea salt to your water. Questions about which electrolytes to buy? I'll explain electrolyte supplements in more detail in the Intuitive Fasting Toolbox in chapter 10.

Exercise on your non-fasting days: No matter what type of exercise you're doing—it could be anything from training for a triathlon to taking a 20-minute walk in your neighborhood—do it before your first meal on your non-fasting days. This way, you're not pushing your body to work out after you've been fasting for 20 to 22 hours, and any post-workout hunger will happen during your feeding window.

Consider incorporating MCT oil into your routine: MCT (medium-chain triglyceride) oil is a high-quality fat made from coconuts. MCT oil can help you deepen your ketosis because your body can quickly convert medium-chain triglycerides, the fats that make up MCT oil, into usable energy for your cells. MCTs are particularly helpful when taken before a workout—and even better when mixed with coffee or tea.[3] Although optional, you can start with 1 teaspoon a day and increase to as many as 4 teaspoons a day.

The Benefits of Your Almost-OMAD Fast

The longer we fast, the more we put our bodies under higher amounts of the positive stress we learned about in chapter 3. As a result, mechanisms buried deep within your body start to kick into gear. More specifically, your cells launch an adaptive stress response (remember our friend, hormesis?), which includes increasing their expression of antioxidant defenses, protein quality control, DNA repair, increase in stem cells, mitochondrial biogenesis, downregulation of inflammation, and autophagy—just to name a few.[4] In short, think of this week as your own, personal accelerated, anti-aging treatment.

Unlike decreased hunger, balanced blood sugar, and increased energy, you won't necessarily feel these positive shifts happening in your body in real time; the good news is that they still have an enormous impact on your long-term health and even on your ability to prevent disease. This week we're focusing on the hidden benefits of fasting—the ones you can't see or feel today but that will no doubt improve your long-term health and quality of life drastically. So while the claims you see online that fasting can "make you live longer" or "prevent disease" might seem crazy at first, in this chapter you'll learn the science and understand that, actually, they're not far-fetched at all.

Disease Prevention

It's clear that fasting has a lot of potential in terms of preventing age-related diseases. But what about illnesses that affect us no matter what our age? The research in this area has blown up in recent years as well, so brace yourself, because there's a lot to cover.

Both animal and human research has shown that intermittent fasting can improve risk factors for a wide range of chronic diseases, including autoimmune and inflammatory diseases, neurodegenerative diseases, chronic pain, and even cancer.

Studies on intermittent fasting have revealed its ability to improve a wide range of inflammation-related diseases, including autoimmune diseases like multiple sclerosis (MS), fibromyalgia, and rheumatoid arthritis. One study showed that fasting reduced MS-like symptoms by changing the makeup of the gut microbiome, and another showed that a fasting-mimicking diet given to mice reduced the clinical severity of MS in all of them and actually completely reversed MS symptoms in 20 percent of them.[5, 6]

We have already learned that fasting can fend off chronic inflammation, which means it may protect against inflammation-related diseases like psoriasis, asthma, and irritable bowel syndrome (IBS). These types of diseases occur when the immune system gets overzealous and starts to launch an inflammatory immune response in the body. Intermittent fasting may be able to quell an overactive immune system without affecting its ability to respond to real threats, like bacteria and viruses. In fact, in a study published in the journal *Cell*, researchers discovered that fasting reduces inflammation and improves chronic inflammatory diseases without affecting the immune system's response to acute infections.[7]

Another incredibly exciting area of research has to do with fasting's potential role in reducing the risk of developing cancer. For example, fasting for more than 13 hours per night was linked to a decreased risk of breast cancer recurrence.[8] The authors of the study concluded that fasting may represent a simple nonpharmacologic strategy for this reduction and suspect the connection is due to fasting's ability to improve blood sugar regulation and sleep. Another possible explanation may be that fasting assists the body in clearing out toxins and damaged cells.[9]

Researchers have also studied fasting as a possible complementary treatment to increase the efficacy of chemotherapy and reduce its many side effects.[10] For example, the authors of a small but significant study wrote: "10 patients who fasted in combination with chemotherapy reported that fasting was not only feasible and safe but caused a reduction in a wide range of side effects accompanied by an apparently normal and possibly aug-

mented chemotherapy efficacy."[11] This is a big deal, considering the fact that chemotherapy side effects can be extremely severe.

The science on cancer cells and fasting is fascinating. Many types of cancer cells are famously reliant on sugar and are extremely vulnerable to nutrient deprivation. So, when you have your body switch to burning fat, cancerous cells suffer because they cannot effectively fuel themselves. Essentially, by fasting before or during chemotherapy, you are allowing the drug to target cancer cells more effectively while protecting your own cells at the same time.

When talking about preventing and treating disease, I'd be remiss if I didn't mention brain health. Why? Because so many of us suffer not only from mental health issues like anxiety, depression, obsessive-compulsive disorder (OCD), and post-traumatic stress disorder (PTSD), but also from autoimmune brain diseases like Alzheimer's and MS. Not to mention that many of us feel sluggish and foggy-brained and have trouble concentrating on a daily basis. Brain issues are an epidemic. Depression is the leading cause of disability worldwide, and anxiety disorders affect more than 40 million Americans. Why this catastrophic rise in brain problems? In recent years, science may have uncovered an answer that could explain the one common factor among many of these otherwise highly differentiated cases: an inflammatory immune response in the brain.

Autoimmune conditions themselves have also grown to epidemic proportions in our lifetimes, affecting an estimated 50 million Americans. Autoimmune disease attacks the body's own tissues in an overzealous attempt to slay invaders like viruses or bacteria, and frequently targets specific areas of the body—the brain included.

Millions of people's immune systems are at war with their brains and nervous tissue, and this particular problem is drastically underdiagnosed. Autoimmune-inflammatory brain issues like multiple sclerosis, Parkinson's, Alzheimer's, and autism are affecting people now more than ever before in human history.

So what gives? Well, just like diabetes or heart disease, all the conditions I just mentioned are intricately connected to our lifestyles and the negative effect our lifestyles have on our inflammation levels.

New research is looking at how inflammation can damage the brain's protective blood-brain barrier (BBB).[12] The blood-brain barrier is the barrier that keeps substances—including many harmful ones, like toxins and inflammatory signals—from traveling from the bloodstream into the brain. The BBB isn't super-well understood, but what we do know is that issues like chronic stress and depression are associated with a loss of the integrity of the BBB, which means it becomes leaky and allows substances to pass through.[13]

It is possible that this could lead to brain problems such as those now often referred to as neurological autoimmunity. This loss of blood-brain barrier integrity can overactivate the brain's immune microglia cells, which are cells that can act as the cleaning system in the central nervous system and trigger an inflammatory autoimmune response. In other words, people's immune systems might be attacking their brains and nervous tissue in response to inflammation that could have started somewhere else entirely, such as in the gut. When in balance, microglial cells act like the brain's housecleaning team, tidying up and making sure the nervous system is working optimally. When overactivated by something like "leaky brain syndrome" or a loss of BBB integrity, the housecleaning team goes into an inflammatory attack mode.

There's strong preclinical evidence that fasting can prevent and slow down the progression of extremely prevalent conditions like Alzheimer's disease and Parkinson's disease. It does this by increasing the ability of brain cells to resist stress and stimulate autophagy, boosting mitochondrial function, antioxidant defenses, increasing stem cells, and DNA repair, according to a study published in the *New England Journal of Medicine*. Some researchers think that because ketones are a more efficient energy source than glucose, they may protect against age-related decline in the central nervous system that might cause dementia and other brain-related illnesses. Also, as I have mentioned earlier, fasting increases the levels of brain-derived neurotrophic factor (BDNF) and supports neuroplasticity, your brain's ability to make new neurons. BDNF plays a role in preventing neurodegenerative disease, but researchers are also studying it for the role it may have in managing chronic pain. This all makes sense, considering the fact that inflammation is a factor in both brain disease and chronic pain.

Conventional thought likes to separate mental health from physical health. In reality, mental health *is* physical health. Our brain is part of our body, and there are measurable physiological implications that can drive brain health problems. We often think of mental health conditions as a "chemical imbalance," but inflammation may actually be the underlying driver of any subsequent imbalance. Inflammation has the potential to trigger depression, exacerbate it, and even be its root cause. As the authors of a study showed, while there are many factors that affect mental health, increased inflammatory activation in the nervous system is a known factor.[14] And do you want to know what's even more shocking? Antidepressants have been shown to decrease inflammation, so that may be an unknown mechanism by which they help improve mood.

Depression was the first disorder to be linked to inflammation and autoimmunity, but anxiety, PTSD, and panic disorders soon followed. For example, one study showed that people with lupus have higher levels of anxiety due to inflammation in the brain.[15] Research has shown that anxiety symptoms are correlated with increased levels of inflammatory cytokines, which are inflammatory substances secreted by immune cells.

In the research on mental health conditions and inflammation, inflammatory cytokines come up again and again. In fact, there's even a concept called the cytokine model of cognitive function, which says that cytokines play an important role in cognitive processes at the molecular level, and that learning, memory, mood, and attention may all be disrupted by processes that are mediated by cytokines. In other words, cytokine status has the potential to sabotage brain health, mental health, and so much more. This is important in the context of this book because fasting has been shown in research studies to decrease levels of pro-inflammatory cytokines, like IL-1β, IL-6, and tumor necrosis factor α.[16]

Another theory out there has to do with mitochondria, which we've already learned quite a bit about when we talked about energy production and fatigue. Well, studies also suggest an intriguing link between depression and mitochondrial diseases. Our mitochondria are the cellular powerhouses of our cells, but they also help regulate brain function.

Scientists suspect that alteration in mito-chondrial function may increase oxidative stress and apoptosis (cell death) and ultimately cause depressive symptoms. This is important for you and me in the context of this book, because a huge part of becoming metabolically flexible is re-teaching the mitochondria to rely on both fat and sugar for fuel, which helps create healthier and more productive mitochondria. This could theoretically assist in reversing the underlying causes of depression, too.

Week 3 Goals

The main goal of this week is to complete at least three 20- to 22-hour fasts and to get as deeply into ketosis, hormesis, and autophagy as possible. If you accomplish this, you are able to give your body ade-quate space and time to repair itself on a fundamental cellular level—something that can happen only during times of extended fasting. We spent Weeks 1 and 2 establishing metabolic flexibility, and in Week 3 we are really putting it to the test.

To be able to complete these long fasts, make sure you have additional elec-trolytes (such as a little Himalayan sea salt in water) and plenty of water in general to support your body's newfound metabolic flexibility. If you have any trouble com-pleting the longer fasts this week, make sure you practice mindfulness-based stress reduction, which I'll talk more about

in the Intuitive Fasting Toolbox in chapter 10. Keeping your mind calm this week is critical; completing a 22-hour fast when you're a ball of stress will not aid your health. Eating only within such a short window may also bring up feelings of anxiety—this is normal. Remember when I asked you to commit to throwing out the food rules and stepping out of your com-fort zone? This is where that really comes in. This week you are truly abandoning what you thought you knew about meal-times and eating, and instead you are get-ting back to the basics of what your body genuinely needs and what it can do.

Let me be clear: this is no easy feat at first. You may initially feel isolated or won-der "Why the heck am I doing this again?" If you experience these feelings, remem-ber that you are chasing real, science-backed benefits like increased resilience against disease and increased longevity and cellular renewal. Longer fasts are all about long-term benefits and improving the health of the future you, who wants to be free of age-related diseases and decline. Obviously, in this 4-Week Flexi-ble Fasting Plan we are doing only a few of these long fasts over the course of Week 3, which is not going to be enough to fully prevent future disease or extend longevity. The point of Week 3 is to lean your body into these healing fasts so that you can make intermittent 20-plus-hour fasts a staple part of your lifestyle going forward.

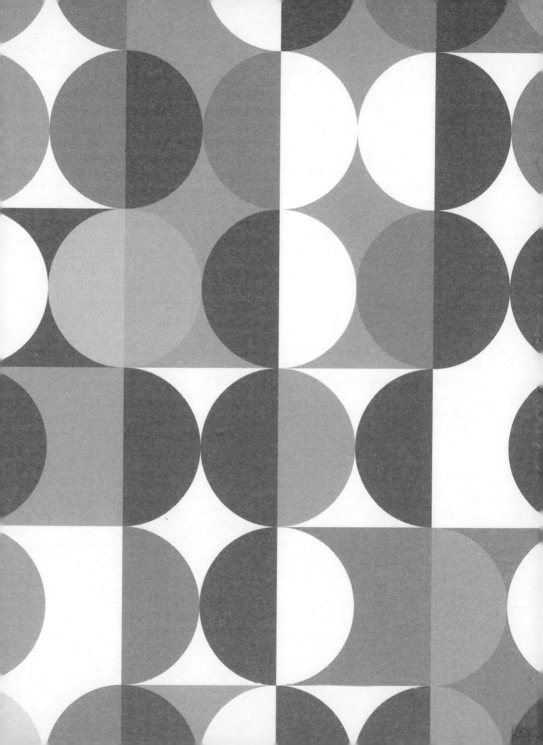

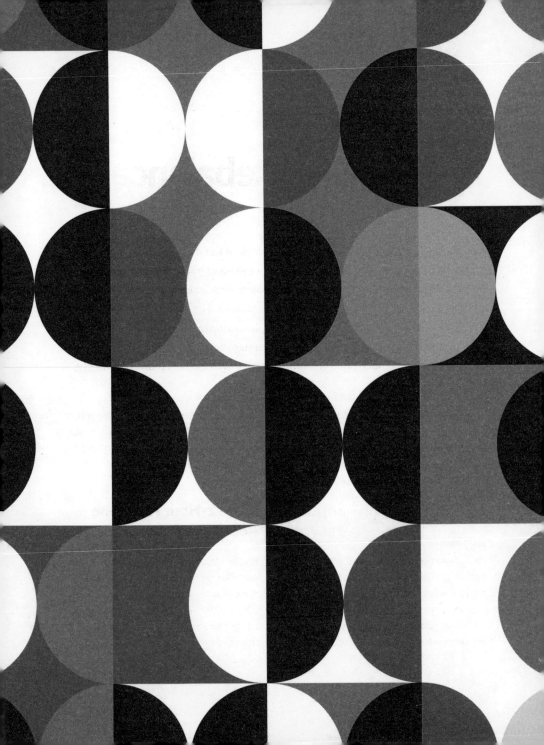

CHAPTER 8

Week 4: Rebalance

Congratulations! You've reached the final week of the 4-Week Flexible Fasting Plan. You completed some pretty long fasts last week—and your body is now adapted to burn both sugar and fat for fuel like an absolute pro. So far in the 4-Week Flexible Fasting Plan, you've put your body to the test and asked it to adapt to changes in macronutrient intake and fasting windows. In response, your body has done exactly what it was designed to do: rise to the challenge. You may even feel shocked and impressed by how much stronger and adaptable your body is than you thought.

For this final week, we're turning our attention to our hormones. Why? Because one of the most important things to know about your body is that every part is connected, and your hormones are responsible for weaving every system together. They act as messengers, sending instructions to different areas of your body and regulating everything from your mood to your digestion to your metabolism—like a beautiful interconnected dance between every system of your body. You want your hormones to be happy because, at the end of the day, they're often what makes the difference between your being happy or not. Hormones also play a key role in your ability to access your intuition about food, which is the second thing we'll be focusing on this week.

The 12-Hour Hormone Rebalance Fast

For this final stretch of the 4-Week Flexible Fasting Plan, we'll be returning to the original 12-hour eating window from Week 1. But now, in Week 4, we will be experimenting with more Clean Carb-Up days than you may have done in Week 2.

On Week 2 the Clean Carb-Up days were optional, but I would like you to experiment with moderating your clean carbohydrates for 2 to 4 days this week. The goal here is to figure out what the most sustainable macronutrient ratio will be for you in the long term by discovering your carb sweet spot. In other words, we're experimenting with different carbohydrate intakes to find an amount you can aim to continue with long after the 4-Week Flexible Fasting Plan has come to an end.

You might be wondering why we'd be doing shorter fasts for the last week of the plan. Shouldn't we be increasing our fasting time even more than last week to increase the benefits?

Actually, no. I've designed the 4-Week Flexible Fasting Plan to allow you to stretch and contract your daily eating windows to help you become metabolically flexible, *sustainably*. If diet variability is a yoga class for your metabolism, then Rebalance Week is the Savasana. This tailored approach allows you to use both the tools of fasting and a low-carb diet to help you reconnect with the way your body was supposed to feel. The Cellular Renewal fasts in Week 3 allowed you to put some sustainably burning firewood on the fire. Week 4 is all about putting some clean kindling on top to see what the perfect combination is. Metabolic flexibility is about balance and the ability to burn both glucose and fat when you want to.

To find your right carbohydrate intake, you'll rely on signs from your body and that good ol' intuition that I've mentioned so many times throughout this book. Many of you will feel totally energized and in harmony with your body while eating a low-carb, high-fat diet. After an initial adjustment period, many people feel great eating low-carb and staying in ketosis over the long term but still could benefit from some occasional conservative carb cycling every now and then.

In contrast, many of you do best with the Cyclical Ketotarian approach you may have experimented with in Week 2, so we'll continue to learn about, and experiment with, Clean Carb Cycling this week. So, 3 to 5 days during your Rebalance week will be a 12:12 fasting-to-eating window, focusing on the fasting-mimicking benefits of a Ketotarian diet, as you did in Week 1. For example:

Breakfast: Zucchini-Asparagus Hash **–8:00 a.m.**

Lunch: Curried Tuna Salad Wraps **–12:00 p.m.**

Snack: Creamy Herb Veggie Dip with red bell pepper strips –2:30 p.m.

Dinner: Walnut Portobellos in Sage Butter –7:00 p.m.

The difference in Week 4 is that the remaining 2 to 4 days can be Clean Carb Up days, which means increasing your *net carb* intake from 55 grams or fewer to somewhere between 75 and 150 grams.

Cyclical Ketotarian: Clean Carb-Up Days

The fact is, we are all different, and while some people do really well in long-term nutritional ketosis, others experience a greater benefit (and gain metabolic flexibility) when they strategically cycle out of ketosis now and then by upping their intake of healthy carbs. If you felt way better on your Clean Carb-Up days in Week 2, it may be because you simply need more carbs to balance things out in your body.

Let me be clear: needing more clean carbs is not a bad thing. You're already familiar with carb-up days, but in this chapter, we'll learn more about the benefits of carbohydrates. Gasp! Yes, you read that correctly. I'm going to talk about the benefits of carbohydrates. Contrary to popular belief and the wellness industry's tendency to villainize particular nutrients (*cough, cough,* the low-fat, zero-fat, no-fat-ever diet craze in the 1980s), there is no macronutrient that is fundamentally bad across the board. Carbs can be helpful macronutrients. As long as they're eaten in a way that is healthy and that works for your biochemistry, they provide great fuel for your body and help many of your hormones and brain neurotransmitters function at optimal capacity.

Your body actually makes some sugar through a process called gluconeogenesis, even when you aren't consuming any carbohydrates (like in Week 1 and Week 3), but sometimes some additional clean carbs from our food can give our bodies that extra boost. There is a time and place for some kindling on the fire, even when you have that firewood of fat-burning burning bright.

So, how do you know if you need more carbs in your life in the long term? You should consider leaning into the Clean Carb-Up days if you've experienced any of the following during the previous 3 weeks:

- You feel amped, wired, or anxious more than usual.

- You've experienced changes in your menstrual cycle length or PMS symptoms.

- You're having trouble sleeping or winding down at night.

- You feel cranky, irritable, and more easily frustrated than usual.

- You're experiencing heart palpitations or a racing heart.

- Your hunger signals still don't feel in balance—you're unsatisfied and hungry all the time.

- You're noticing exacerbated thyroid symptoms such as hair loss or fatigue.

If you've noticed any restlessness, insomnia, anxiety, menstrual cycle changes, or hunger during these first three weeks, don't worry. That can happen as you shift your metabolism from being just a sugar-burner to becoming more keto- or fat-adapted. But since we are all different, you can experiment with Clean Carb-Up days this week and in the long term. That way, you can have the best of both worlds: by increasing your carbohydrate intake in a strategic way, you can enjoy the benefits of fasting and ketosis without sacrificing your hormone balance.

So how do you do Cyclical Ketotarian this week? On your regular Ketotarian days, your diet has consisted of fewer than 55 grams of net carbs per day. This week you can experiment with adding in more carbs, which means increasing your intake to 75 to 150 grams of net carbs up to 4 days a week. The Clean Carb-Up days can be consecutive or mixed throughout the week. Here's what a 12:12 Clean Carb-Up day might look like:

Breakfast: Avocado + Grapefruit with Coconut Topping –8:00 a.m.

Lunch: Minted Chickpea Salad –12:00 p.m.

Snack: Spicy Almond Butter Dip with cucumber slices and a Pineapple Smoothie –2:30 p.m.

Dinner: Spinach-Artichoke Turmeric Rice –7:00 p.m.

Compared with the number of carbs you've been eating on the low-carb days, this might seem like a *lot* of carbs. What about everything we just learned about the negative effect of carbs on our metabolism, blood sugar, and inflammation levels? Well, the truth is, even the upper limit of 150 grams of net carbs on your Clean Carb-Up day is by no means high-carb compared with the standard Western diet. In fact, most American diets consist of somewhere between 45 and 65 percent carbohydrates, which if you're calculating using a 2,000-calorie diet, comes out to somewhere between 200 to 300 net carbs per day. This is significantly more than 150 grams of net carbs, especially when you consider the fact that, in most cases, people are eating these carbs in the form of soda, white sugar, white bread, and other refined carbohydrates that damage their health in other ways as well. This is another reason why you should not beat yourself up if you discover that you thrive better when you're eating more carbs. The type of carbs you eat matters; not all carbs are created equal.

The explanation for why some people need more carbs than others isn't a simple one. The truth is, we don't know everything there is to know about why some people need more carbs to thrive. Ketones are amazing substances with the ability to reduce inflammation and oxidative stress and bring balance back to insulin and other hormones when used correctly. And most of the time, ketosis can actually help hormone imbalances. But for some people, long-term ketosis can also put stress (not the good kind) on the body and exacerbate hormone issues, especially those involving female sex hormones, sleep, and weight management. And if there's one thing we know for sure, it's that if one hormone is out of balance, it can throw off your whole body.

Clean-Carb Cycling: For Sleep, Sex Hormones, and Stalled Goals

Even though your body was brilliantly making its own sugar through gluconeogenesis during your regular Ketotarian foods and fasting, consuming additional carbohydrates every now and then can be a great tool to signal to the body that it's not in fasting mode. This can maintain your hormone and neurotransmitter balance, which has beneficial consequences for what I call the "3 S's" for Clean Carb Cycling: sleep, sex hormones, and stalled goals.

Sleep

If your sleeping patterns shifted on a low-carb diet, you're not alone. Some people report that they have trouble winding down for bed or wake up at 2 or 3 a.m. with their minds racing. Scientists are still trying to figure out exactly why this occurs,

but we know that all of our hormones are interconnected, so it helps to look at this phenomenon from a holistic perspective.

Let's start with the adrenal glands. We already know about the stress response, chronic stress and HPA (brain-adrenal) axis dysfunctions. Well, if it's not done correctly, a long-term ketogenic diet can have a negative impact on your brain-adrenal axis, or communication line. The consequence of this is an imbalance in cortisol, your main stress hormone.

You might be wondering what this has to do with sleep. Well, your sleep-wake cycle is regulated by two hormones: cortisol and melatonin. In the morning, your cortisol level is higher. It causes a healthy type of stress that makes you feel alert, active, and helps you get up and out of bed. After its peak in the morning, cortisol declines throughout the day. As cortisol declines, melatonin—also known as your sleep hormone—starts to increase, peaking in the evening when it gets dark. When melatonin peaks, it makes you feel sleepy, groggy, and relaxed enough to fall off to sleep.

If you disrupt your cortisol production by stressing your HPA axis, your melatonin also gets confused and you may have trouble getting to sleep.

This is particularly true if your HPA axis was already fatigued at the start of this plan, which we learned in chapter 6, is extremely common. If that's the case, long-term ketosis can make you feel

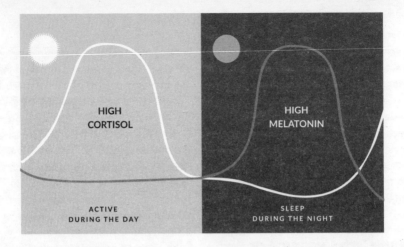

HIGH
CORTISOL

HIGH
MELATONIN

ACTIVE
DURING THE DAY

SLEEP
DURING THE NIGHT

stressed, anxious, and totally amped when you're trying to get to sleep at night—and then extremely tired throughout the day because melatonin will try to surge at the wrong time. That's all thanks to a disruption in your daily cortisol-melatonin rhythms.

However, HPA axis stress isn't the only possible connection between sleep issues and a long-term low-carb diet. In fact, as it turns out, some carbohydrates are helpful for optimal serotonin production. You've probably heard of serotonin before—it's a neurotransmitter that helps soothe your brain, producing feelings of positivity and relaxation. Serotonin plays a key role in helping you feel calm enough to sleep and preventing negative or anxious thinking, which can definitely keep you up at night staring at the ceiling. When you eat carbohydrates, you release insulin, which helps an amino acid called tryptophan enter the brain. Tryptophan is then

converted into serotonin, where it gets to work making you feel happy and relaxed. This connection is also possibly why, when we start cutting out carbs, some people can feel, for lack of a better word, sad about it. It's also another reason why carbohydrates can be so addictive and why quitting unhealthy carbohydrates can be difficult; they cause a massive surge in insulin and therefore a big boost in serotonin and good feelings.

Are you ready to have your mind blown? Melatonin, your sleepy-time hormone, is actually *made from serotonin*. This means that carbohydrates are helpful for melatonin production, and if you mess with this intricate connection between melatonin, serotonin, and carbohydrates, it may have the unexpected consequence of messing with your sleep.

The good news is that a Cyclical Ketotarian diet is the best way to avoid the potential negative effects of a low-carb fasting diet plan on your serotonin and sleep while still tapping into all the amazing health benefits. By adding in Clean Carb-Up days, you're making sure that your body has some healthy carbohydrates to produce healthy levels of serotonin and melatonin without becoming reliant on quick hits of simple unhealthy, addictive carbs (like refined sugar and refined white flour) to regulate your mood or energy levels. As long as you focus on eating high-quality carbohydrates (like those found in sweet potatoes, fruit, and rice)—and only eat them in moderation and intermittently—carbs can be extremely helpful for your sleep quality.

Sex Hormones

You may have read or heard that women should not try intermittent fasting because it can interfere with their hormone balance. Admittedly, there is *some* truth to this. The way sex hormones behave is extremely complicated, but, essentially, the brain-ovary axis (also known as the hypothalamic-pituitary-gonadal, or HPG, axis) is your brain's line of communication with your ovaries. Your brain speaks by sending hormones, which are basically chemical emails, to the ovaries. This then prompts your ovaries to release estrogen and progesterone. A healthy HPG axis is essential for you to feel great on a daily basis and also plays a major role in fertility and pregnancy.

When it comes to intermittent fasting, women do seem to be more sensitive than men. This is, at least in part, due to the fact that women have more kisspeptin, a neuropeptide that stimulates the hypothalamus.[1] Research suggests that these higher kisspeptin levels in women can cause the HPG axis to get thrown out of sorts, and, as a result, women miss their periods, develop PMS symptoms, or just feel generally "off" hormonally. This could, in theory, impact fertility as well as metabolism in some women, although more studies need to be done.

Interestingly, other research shows that fasting might actually be easier—and more beneficial—for women. For example, studies have actually demonstrated that adrenaline burns more fat in women than men, which likely has to do with women's higher average percentage of body fat. Typically, essential body fat is 3 percent of body mass for men and 12 percent of body mass for women; and, on average, women typically have 6 to 11 percent more body fat than men.[2] Women also burn more fat, fewer carbohydrates, and less protein than men at the same exercise intensity.

However, no two women are exactly alike. Clinically, I find that some women do great with longer intermittent fasting windows—many of my patients report that it has helped with irregular cycles, cramps, and even hormonal acne—and some do better with lighter fasting windows and more of a Cyclical Ketotarian approach. Does this mean that women who are sensitive to intermittent fasting shouldn't do it at all? No. For these individuals, it may just require some more gentle fasting windows and some Clean Carb-Up days to be added to their long-term lifestyle plan.

So how do you clean-carb cycle for better sex hormone balance?

Many of my patients also do quite well when they increase their carb intake around their periods and ovulation—once or twice a month—as opposed to cycling in added carbs every week. Here's what to do:

- On days 1 and 2 of your menstrual cycle, increase your carbs.

- You can also try increasing your carb intake after ovulation, around days 19 and 20 of your menstrual cycle, which is about 5 days after ovulation. You can experiment with this and see how you feel.

As you experiment, pay close attention to energy, mood, and PMS symptoms and keep in mind that not everyone's cycle is the same. Feel free to play around with which days you decide to increase your carbs. This simple adjustment is often all you need to get rid of any potential hormonal side effects of fasting and a low-carb eating plan. During your 4-Week Flexible Fasting Plan, feel free to move your Clean Carb-Up days according to your cycle. Also, if you find that you feel better eating more clean carbs when you break your fasts, add in more Clean Carb-Up days during any of the 4-week eating windows, even on Weeks 1 and 3.

Stalled Goals

Weight loss plateaus are very irritating and unfortunately are common. I often have patients come to me and say they have tried everything. And whether they are trying to lose a lot of weight or just those last few pounds, plateaus can be extremely frustrating. No one likes to spin their wheels—what's the point of a healthy lifestyle if it doesn't pay off?

Stalled weight loss goals can happen for any number of reasons, but since we've already learned about the relationship between serotonin and carbohydrates, we'll start there. Serotonin doesn't just help you produce melatonin for great sleep, it also helps regulate appetite. In fact, this neurotransmitter has been nicknamed "nature's appetite suppressant" because of its ability to curb hunger and cravings by making you feel satiated. When you cut carbohydrates too low for too long, you run the risk of dropping serotonin to a place where you start to feel hungry all the time. This can make it extremely difficult to lose weight.

Speaking of hunger, I want to talk about leptin in this section on weight loss resistance. As we learned earlier in the book, leptin is a hormone produced by fat cells that helps suppress appetite, signaling to your body that it has enough fat stored and your body doesn't need to eat any more. If you are overweight or have chronic inflammation, your leptin levels can stay chronically high and this can interfere with leptin signaling. Leptin resistance causes the brain to think it's starving when in reality it's not. This causes the body to stubbornly hold on to weight. That's why, for many people, one of the major benefits of this fasting plan will be its ability to lower leptin levels and help you feel more satiated.

Sounds great, right?

Unfortunately, leptin levels fluctuate according to such a complex feedback loop that lowering them long-term can also go awry. This is especially true if you're part of a certain group, which typically includes those who do not have leptin resistance in the first place, those who are at a healthy weight at the start of the 4-Week Flexible Fasting Plan, or those who are generally lean but have maybe a few pounds they'd like to lose. In these people, a long-term, low-carb eating plan can lead to leptin levels that decline so much they cause your body to think that fat stores are too low and that you need to eat—*stat*. When this happens, your hunger signals tell your body that it's in starvation mode and you need to be conserving fat instead of burning it. Cue: significantly stalled goals. Remember, bal-ance is everything. We don't want leptin levels too high, and we don't want leptin levels too low indefinitely, either.

As we already know, disruptions in leptin levels can have various downstream effects in the body. Leptin is intricately connected to other hormones, such as sex hormones like estrogen and proges-terone, thyroid hormones, and even sleep hormones. The good news is that with Clean Carb-Up days, you allow leptin to balance out so you feel satiated and your body doesn't enter starvation mode. This, with the combination of a low-carb diet on other days, which keeps your insulin and leptin sensitivity optimized, will mean that you feel incredible. You'll get the best of both worlds: the leptin-balancing benefits of healthy carbs in moderation, without the leptin-disrupting effects of too many or too few carbs for too long. Clean-Carb Cycling's ability to regulate leptin and ghrelin make it an excellent option for weight loss, especially if you've hit a weight loss plateau or you have just a few stubborn last pounds hanging around.[3, 4]

There's one more type of hormone imbalance we should talk about while we mention stalled goals, and it has to do with the thyroid gland. Thyroid hormone problems can occur for a multitude of reasons, and there are a ton of different types of thyroid issues. For example, you can have autoimmune thyroid problems like Hashimoto's disease; thyroid conver-sion issues like low T3 syndrome; thyroid resistance, which is similar to insulin resistance; and thyroid problems that are secondary to brain-thyroid (hypothalamic-pituitary-thyroid, or HPT) axis dysfunction.

It's hard to give you hard-and-fast rules about how fasting and a low-carb diet will impact your thyroid, and that's largely because thyroid hormones play a role in basically every aspect of your health, including appetite, energy levels, mood, temperature regulation, and sex drive—and an imbalance in thyroid health can cause a wide range of health problems. Many people have thyroid issues; low thyroid function, or hypothyroidism, affects around 20 million Americans, and 1 in 8 women will experience a thyroid issue in her lifetime. And many thyroid problems go undiagnosed or are misdiagnosed as other disorders, so it's impossible to know just how many people suffer from a thyroid issue. It's also impossible to predict how such a wide range of disorders of the thyroid pathway will respond to intermittent fasting and a low-carb diet.

That said, by and large, long-term low-carb diets and fasting have been shown to lower thyroid hormone levels. For some people, this can slow down thyroid production and conversion and increase symptoms like low sex drive, low energy, and weight loss resistance.

For others, the health benefits of fasting and low-carb living seem to outweigh any potential thyroid hormone dip. In this group, the body is able to function at optimal capacity even though it has less thyroid hormone available. I often see patients who fast regularly and eat a healthy fat-based Ketotarian diet and have slightly lower T3 thyroid levels but feel great, because, like a hybrid car, they are more efficient with their energy. Carbs are often thought to increase the thyroid hormone T3, which may be a component to some people's T3 levels, but carbs also increase the ability of T3 to handle the glucose in the blood. During the 4-Week Flexible Fasting Plan, you'll have less glucose in your blood in general, which means you'll naturally need less T3. When you become more keto- or fat-adapted and metabolically flexible, imagine your metabolism becoming like a hybrid vehicle and less of a gas-guzzling SUV.

So what should you do if you have a diagnosed thyroid issue? I'd recommend getting your thyroid levels tested before and after the 4-Week Flexible Fasting Plan to see how low-carb eating and fasting affect your thyroid levels. But even more important, pay close attention to your symptoms throughout the plan. If you're experiencing an exacerbation of your thyroid symptoms, definitely focus on incorporating the Clean Carb-Up days throughout the plan. If you feel amazing, keep up with what you're doing—even if your thyroid test comes back and your levels are a little low. At the end of the day, in my practice, I use how someone feels and the full context of their health as the ultimate determinants of how much thyroid hormones they need.

Clean Carb Cycling is the ideal way to push past a weight loss plateau or stalled goals, and I often recommend it to my patients. There is one exception, though. I don't typically recommend the higher range of this option (150 grams of net carbs per day) for people with insulin resistance, diabetes, or inflammatory issues or people who have more than 10 pounds of weight they want to lose. If you have one of these issues, you are more likely to be more sensitive to carbohydrates. With that said, you can definitely still experiment with a Cyclical Ketotarian approach, as we are all different, with many unique variables.

A final tip of Clean Carb Cycling: experiment with increasing your carbohydrate intake on your more intense workout days (well, if you have those). Higher-carb days help your body refuel muscle glycogen, which studies have shown can help reduce muscle breakdown and may even improve athletic performance.[5] With a Cyclical Ketotarian approach, you're able to fuel high-intensity exercise while also burning fat on low-carb days. In other words, you're teaching your body how to burn fat while also getting all the important hormone-supporting benefits of carbs.

Week 4 Goals

As you experiment with Clean Carb-Up days, assess your energy, brain function, digestion, sleep, and overall life enjoyment. The real goal of this week is to be fine with whatever you uncover. You may find that you thrive in long-term low-carb land, which is something I often observe in insulin- or weight loss–resistant folks and those with insatiable cravings or neurological problems.

You may find the opposite.·

If you feel better with higher carbohydrate intake, there should be no shame in that. A lot of people beat themselves up or feel like they've failed if they go over an arbitrary "carb limit" they've set for themselves, but, really, it's all about what works for you. In fact, a lot of women actually do really well with slightly higher carb intake. And if you're an athlete, boosting your carb intake before a big workout or event can be helpful as well. Ultimately, this week is about experimenting and tweaking your fasting plan and macronutrient ratio until you find what helps you reach your goals in a balanced, sustainable way.

Once you do that, you'll have truly reconnected with your intuition about food—and you'll be well on your way to finding peace with food.

PART THREE

Intuitive Fasting: Getting Started and Beyond

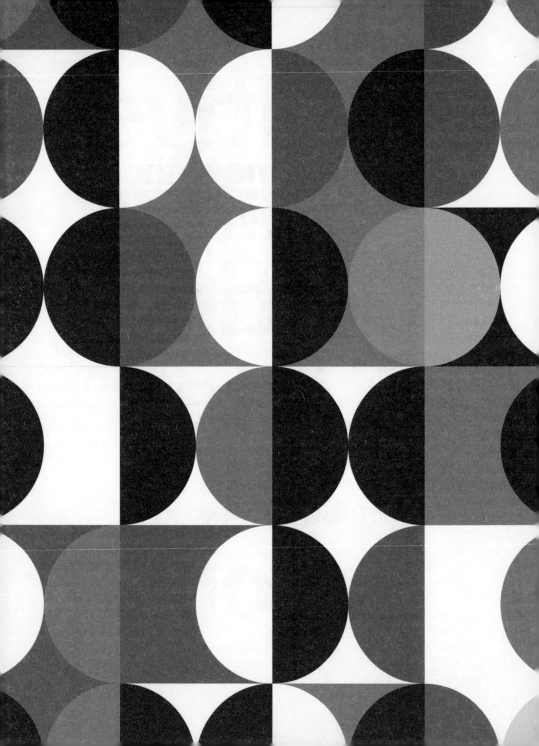

CHAPTER 9

Welcome to the Ketotarian Lifestyle

In this chapter, I'll introduce you to a basic Ketotarian eating guide, which will be the foundation of your diet for the 4-Week Flexible Fasting Plan. This includes many vegan-keto, vegetarian-keto, and pescatarian-keto (or what I call Vegaquarian) options. Then I'll show you how to adapt your Ketotarian plan to your tastes and habits, which means adding in some omnivore options like grass-fed beef and organic chicken if you'd like some more flexibility with your protein options. (I call this Ketotarian-Vegavore.) I'll show you exactly which foods to add to your diet during your Clean Carb-Up days and exactly how to break your fast for optimal digestion and blood sugar balance. Finally, I'll talk about not just what to eat but how to eat by introducing my thoughts on mindful eating and overeating.

Ketotarian Days: What to Eat

Welcome to Ketotarian land! Here is where we dig into all the delicious, nutrient-dense, filling foods you get to eat on your plant-centric ketogenic diet plan. This is a book about intermittent fasting, but, honestly, this might just be the most important chapter, so pay close attention!

Remember, on days and weeks when I instruct you to follow a Ketotarian diet, what I mean in terms of macronutrients is:

- 60 to 75 percent of your calories should come from fat (but it can be more!).

- 15 to 30 percent of your calories should come from protein.

- 5 to 15 percent of your calories should from carbohydrates.

Fats, proteins, and vegetables will be the foundation of your diet on your Ketotarian days, so I've outlined the healthiest sources of each on the following pages. These are the foods you should be stocking up on—and eating plenty of—during the 4-Week Flexible Fasting Plan.

The ultimate goal for your new Ketotarian lifestyle is to make sure you are eating quality and healing, clean keto foods. However, it is very important to find the right ratios of macronutrients that will help you become fat-adapted and enhance how you feel. There are plenty of keto food-tracking apps that you can download easily to your smartphone. Keto diet-logging apps make it simple, tracking how much fat, protein, and carbs you have eaten and how much you need for the day. So, put that calculator and pencil away and use technology to your advantage. And, remember, once you get the hang of it, this will be second nature. You will know what your body loves, hates, and needs in order to thrive.

Food-logging apps are not meant to make you become obsessive about food, but to help you grow your awareness of what you are eating. Some people find that food tracking long-term is helpful,

while others don't need to once they get the hang of what their body loves and where they feel the best. Once you become aware of the macronutrients in your food (where your fuel is coming from), the goal is to just eat until satiety—in other words, until you're satisfied, not until you're overly full.

If the healthy foods on the Ketotarian food list are new to you, give yourself grace and patience. One option for you is to ease into things. Spend the first two weeks of the 4-Week Flexible Fasting Plan just eating from the allowed food list. Don't worry too much about the serving sizes or tracking your macronutrients—just eat from the foods on the allowed list until you're satisfied. Don't log your food intake for these 2 weeks if you don't want to; just keep it simple and eat within the specific eating window of the week that you are in. Spend these first 2 weeks getting used to these healthy food choices, clearing out your pantry and fridge of anything that isn't on the "allowed list."

Vegan-Keto and Vegetarian-Keto: The Foundation of the Ketotarian Plate

Healthy Fats

Depending on your size and activity level, your fat intake should be about 20 to 40 grams per meal. Focusing on healthy fats and cutting unhealthy carbs to curb cravings is the secret to becoming fat-adapted. This will make you a fat-burning, anti-inflammatory, anti-aging, brain-fueling powerhouse. Fat is your fuel, so let's talk about exactly what kind of fats to buy and incorporate into every meal you eat.

Cooking Oils

The way you use fats matters, and it's important to know the smoking points of the oils you're using. That's why I've divided the good-fat list into those appropriate for cooking and those that should be consumed at room temperature or low heat.

Oils to use for cooking:

- Avocado oil
- Coconut oil
- Grass-fed ghee (clarified butter)
- Hazelnut oil
- Macadamia nut oil
- Olive oil (not virgin or extra-virgin olive oil, which are for room-temperature use)

- Palm fruit oil
- Palm kernel oil
- Dark roasted sesame oil (lower-temperature stir-fries)

Oils and fats to use at room temperature or low heat:

- Unsweetened almond milk yogurt
- Almond oil
- Avocado oil
- Avocados
- Extra-virgin olive oil
- Cocoa butter
- Coconut cream
- Coconut meat
- Full-fat coconut milk
- Unsweetened coconut milk yogurt
- Extra-virgin coconut oil
- Flaxseed oil
- Grass-fed ghee (clarified butter)
- Guacamole
- Hazelnut oil
- Hemp seed oil
- Macadamia nut oil
- MCT oil
- Palm kernel oil
- Walnut oil

Protein

The average optimal protein intake range for a person with 100 pounds of lean body mass would come to 45 to 68 grams per day. Luckily, there are a ton of healthy protein sources to choose from. Here are some of my favorites to make sure you have on hand.

Nuts and Seeds

Nuts are great sources of both fat and protein. Enjoy them solo, on salads, and blended in smoothies, or use them to make nut milks and cheeses. You can also use nut-based flours, like almond or coconut flour, to make your baked goods Ketotarian-friendly.

- **Almonds** (6 grams of protein + 14 grams of fat per 23 nuts)
- **Brazil nuts** (4 grams of protein + 19 grams of fat per 6 nuts)
- **Cashews** (4 grams of protein + 13 grams of fat per 18 nuts)
- **Chia seeds** (4 grams of protein + 9 grams of fat per 2 tablespoons)
- **Flax seeds** (4 grams of protein + 8 grams of fat per 2 tablespoons)
- **Hazelnuts** (4 grams of protein + 17 grams of fat per 21 nuts)
- **Hemp seeds** (11 grams of protein + 13.5 grams of fat per 3 tablespoons)
- **Macadamia nuts** (2 grams of protein + 22 grams of fat per 11 nuts)
- **Pecans** (3 grams of protein + 20 grams fat per 19 nut halves)
- **Pine nuts** (4 grams of protein + 20 grams fat per 165 nuts)
- **Pistachios** (4 grams of protein + 18 grams fat per 49 nuts)
- **Sacha inchi seeds** (9 grams of protein + 16 grams of fat in 40 seeds)
- **Walnuts** (4 grams of protein + 18 grams fat per 14 nut halves)

A word on nuts and seeds: The roughage of nuts and seeds (more so with nuts, less with seeds), as well as the protein lectins and phytates, can irritate some people. In addition, most nuts sold in stores are coated in inflammatory industrial seed oils, like soybean or canola oil. They could also contain partially hydrogenated trans fats, which can contribute to problems as well. Make sure you are going for raw nuts and seeds and properly preparing them. I find that most people do better with soaking nuts and seeds in water overnight to break down the inflammatory lectins and make their nutrients more bioavailable.

Plant-Based Protein

Remember, your Ketotarian plan is high-fat, low-carbohydrate, and moderate protein. In addition to nuts and eggs, here are some plant protein options to bring into your day.

- **Almond butter** (6 grams of protein per ¼ cup butter)

- **Artichokes** (4 grams of protein per ½ cup artichokes)
- **Asparagus** (2.9 grams of protein per 1 cup asparagus)
- **Avocado** (2 grams of protein per ½ avocado)
- **Broccoli** (2 grams of protein per ½-cup serving cooked broccoli)
- **Brussels sprouts** (2 grams of protein per ½ cup sprouts)
- **Hempeh** (tempeh made from hemp seeds) (22 grams of protein per 4 ounces hempeh)
- **Hemp hearts/seeds** (40 grams of protein per 1 cup hemp seeds)
- **Hemp protein powder** (12 grams of protein per 4 tablespoons powder)
- **Maca powder** (3 grams of protein per 1 tablespoon maca powder)
- **Natto** (organic non-GMO) (31 grams of protein per 1 cup natto)
- **Nutritional yeast** (5 grams of protein per 1 tablespoon yeast)
- **Peas** (9 grams of protein per 1 cup cooked peas)
- **Sacha inchi seed protein powder** (24 grams of protein per 4 tablespoons powder)
- **Spinach**: (3 grams of protein per ½-cup serving of cooked spinach)
- **Spirulina** (4 grams of protein per 1 tablespoon spirulina)
- **Tempeh** (organic non-GMO) (31 grams of protein per 1 cup tempeh)

Pasture-Raised Eggs

Eggs are one of my favorite low-key superfoods. This vegetarian-keto option contains about 6 grams of protein and 5 grams of fat per egg. In the past, egg yolks have been criticized, but the reality is, they contain the majority of the egg's nutrients. In fact, I like to think of the egg yolk as nature's multivitamin.

When buying eggs, make sure you're buying the highest quality you can afford. Look for organic, pasture-raised eggs from chickens who roam outside in the sunlight. This will supercharge their nutritional benefits, providing brain foods like choline and omega-3 fats. In fact, pasture-raised eggs have been shown to contain three times more of the brain-beneficial omega-3 fats than supermarket eggs.

Non-Starchy Vegetables

Vegetables are the foundation of your Ketotarian lifestyle over the four weeks of the Flexible Fasting Plan. You should try to fill your plate (minimum of 1 cup) with as many vegetables as you can at each meal. This will make sure you're getting enough fiber—which promotes a diverse healthy gut microbiome—as well as nourishing nutrients to keep your body functioning at optimal capacity.

- Alfalfa sprouts
- Artichokes
- Arugula

- Asparagus
- Bean sprouts
- Beets
- Bok choy
- Broccoli
- Broccoli sprouts
- Brussels sprouts
- Cabbage
- Carrots
- Cauliflower
- Celery
- Chard
- Chives
- Collard greens
- Cucumber
- Dulse
- Eggplant
- Endive
- Ginger
- Jicama
- Kale
- Kelp
- Kohlrabi
- Kombu
- Leeks
- Lettuce
- Mushrooms
- Nori
- Okra
- Olives
- Peppers
- Radishes
- Rhubarb
- Rutabaga
- Scallions
- Seaweed

- Spinach
- Swiss chard
- Turnips
- Water chestnuts

Ketotarian-Vegaquarian: (Mostly) Plant-Based Pescatarian Options

Fish can also be a big piece of the healthy-fat and clean-protein puzzle. The following list contains the cleanest fish on our blue planet, the fish lowest in mercury and other toxins. Aim for about 1 to 2 palm-size portions per meal and focus on the fattier varieties: the ones labeled with two asterisks [**] have the highest healthy omega fats, and the ones labeled with one asterisk [*] have a decent amount of healthy omega fats.

- Alaskan salmon, wild-caught**
- Albacore tuna (U.S./Canada, wild, pole caught)**
- Anchovies**
- Arctic char
- Atlantic mackerel**
- Barramundi
- Bass (saltwater, striped, black)
- Butterfish
- Catfish*
- Clam
- Cod (Alaskan)*
- Crab (Domestic)
- Croaker (Atlantic)
- Flounder*

- Herring**
- Lobster*
- Mahi-mahi (U.S./Ecuador, pole caught)
- Mussels*
- Oysters**
- Pacific halibut*
- Pollock
- Rainbow trout**
- Rockfish*
- Sardines**
- Scallops
- Shrimp*
- Skipjack Tuna (U.S./Canada, wild, pole caught)
- Sole (Pacific)*
- Squid (calamari)
- Tilapia
- Tuna (canned, chunk light)
- Whitefish
- Yellowfin tuna (U.S. Atlantic, wild, pole caught)*
- Yellowfin tuna (Western Central Pacific, wild, hand/line caught)*

Additional Foods and Beverages

In addition to clean protein, healthy fats, and non-starchy vegetables—which should be the foundation of your diet on Ketotarian days—you'll also be permitted small amounts of fruit as well as herbs and Ketotarian-approved beverages. Here's exactly which foods will best sup-port your metabolic flexibility during the Ketotarian days.

Lower-Fructose Fruits

On your regular Ketotarian days, you can enjoy some fruit in moderation. Make sure that your carb amount is 55 grams of net carbs per day or less. Lemons, limes, and berries (and of course the Ketotarian staple avocado) are the best choices as they are the lowest in fruit sugar. On your Clean Carb-Up days you can increase your fruit intake.

- Avocado
- Blackberries
- Blueberries
- Cantaloupe
- Clementine
- Grapefruit
- Honeydew melon
- Kiwi
- Lemons
- Limes
- Oranges
- Papayas
- Passion fruit
- Raspberries
- Rhubarb
- Strawberries
- Tangelos
- Tomatoes

Legumes

As with fruit, legumes such as beans contain some carbs, so they can be used in greater amounts during the Clean Carb-Up days. But just like fruit, they can be used in your baseline Ketotarian days as well, as they are fiber-rich. Just make sure that your net carb amount for the day is 55 grams or fewer. On page 274, I will show you how to pressure-cook legumes to lower the lectin amount and make them more digestible by your body.

- Black beans
- Chickpeas (garbanzo beans)
- Edamame
- Fava beans
- Garbanzo beans
- Great Northern beans
- Green beans
- Kidney beans
- Lentils
- Mung beans
- Navy beans
- Peas
- Pinto beans
- White beans

Herbs

Enjoy fresh or dried herbs as often as you like in whatever quantity you desire. Herbs have amazing healing benefits and can add a lot of flavor to your meals. Add them to salads and stir-fries—you can even incorporate them into your smoothies. You can also find many of these herbs in tea or tincture form, which is another great way to consume them. This is not a complete list, so have at it if something is not listed here:

- Basil
- Bay leaf
- Chili
- Cilantro
- Dill
- Lavender
- Lemon balm
- Mint
- Oregano
- Parsley
- Rosemary
- Sage

Spices

Enjoy fresh or dried in any amount, to taste.

- Allspice
- Anise seed
- Annatto
- Caraway
- Cardamom
- Celery seed
- Cinnamon
- Clove
- Cocoa/cacao
- Coriander
- Cumin
- Fennel
- Fenugreek
- Garlic
- Ginger
- Horseradish
- Juniper
- Juniper berry
- Mace
- Mustard
- Nutmeg
- Paprika
- Peppercorns
- Poppy seeds
- Sea salt
- Sesame seed
- Star anise
- Sumac
- Turmeric
- Vanilla bean (no additives)

Beverages

You might be wondering what kind of beverages you're allowed to consume during your Ketotarian days. Well, here's a list of the low-carb/low-sugar beverages you can stock up on before you start the 4-Week Flexible Fasting Plan:

- Water
- Organic coffee
- Organic tea, including green, white, black, Earl Grey, oolong, and herbal teas
- Carbonated water with no added sweeteners
- Kombucha
- Green juices made only with fresh-pressed green vegetables, lemon, lime, and ginger
- Unsweetened coconut, hemp, macadamia, and almond milk

Low-Carb Natural Sweeteners

Use in small amounts to sweeten things up, to taste.

- Allulose
- Erythritol
- Inulin
- Monk fruit
- Stevia
- Swerve
- Tagatose
- Xylitol

Ketotarian-Vegavore: Clean Omnivore Options

If cutting out chicken and beef sounds like too big a task, especially on top of fasting and removing carbs, then this option is for you. This plan is all about flexibility, and if you want to eat some beef and chicken throughout the 4-Week Flexible Fasting Plan, that's totally okay. In fact, animal protein can get an unfairly bad rap; it's actually full of important nutrients. Grass-fed beef and organ meats contain some of the highest levels of essential nutrients that are necessary for optimal health, such as B vitamins and vitamin A. The 4-Week Flexible Fasting Plan is meant to be exactly as the name says, *flexible,* so I've added grass-fed and organic meats to the protein list, and you can feel free to add these foods.

- Beef
- Bison
- Chicken
- Lamb and mutton
- Organ meats such as liver
- Venison

Just keep in mind that, like eggs, not all meat is raised equally. The conventional meat you typically find in grocery stores is from animals that are fed grains and pumped with hormones, both of which decrease the availability of naturally occurring nutrients and can perpetuate a lot of health problems rather than help overcome them. That's why you should always try to opt for grass-fed, organic, and hormone- and antibiotic-free sources of meat. Support regenerative farms whenever possible.

Cyclical Ketotarian: Clean Carb-Up Days

If you're increasing your carbohydrate intake on certain days—such as during Week 2 and more so in Week 4 of the Flexible Fasting Diet—your diet will look a little different on the cyclical plan described in this section. Welcome to a Cyclical Ketotarian lifestyle. Instead of focusing almost entirely on fats, proteins, and vegetables, you'll be able to increase your intake of fruits, starchy vegetables, and gluten-free grains in order to recalibrate your metabolism during a weight loss plateau, to support sleep issues, or to balance sex hormones.

A couple of days during Week 2 (Recharge) and Week 4 (Rebalance), you'll have the option to increase your carb intake to 75 to 150 grams per day and to reduce your healthy fat intake to compensate for this increase. Ketotarian will still be the foundation of your diet, but you'll be able to add in the following foods in moderation.

Higher-Fructose Fruits

- Apple
- Cherry
- Grape
- Guava
- Lychee
- Mango
- Papaya
- Pear
- Persimmon
- Pineapple
- Quince
- Star fruit
- Watermelon

Starchy Vegetables

- Acorn squash
- Butternut squash
- Peas
- Potatoes
- Sweet potatoes
- Yams

Legumes and Grains

- Black beans
- Edamame
- Fava beans
- Garbanzo beans (chickpeas)
- Great Northern beans
- Green beans
- Kidney beans
- Lentils
- Mung beans
- Navy beans
- Peas
- Pinto beans
- White beans
- Gluten-free oats
- Quinoa
- Rice (white rice is lower in lectins, making it generally more tolerated)

When eating beans, I always recommend soaking them for at least 8 hours before cooking and eating them. Alternatively, you can cook them in a pressure cooker. That will reduce inflammatory compounds often found within these foods and make them easier on your GI tract and better for your microbiome health. I will show you how to pressure-cook beans on page 274.

Sweeteners

- Coconut sugar
- Date syrup
- Honey
- Molasses
- Pure maple syrup
- Rice syrup

What Not to Eat

The 4-Week Flexible Fasting Plan is not about punishing your body or restricting yourself—it's about going for foods that fill you up, reduce inflammation, make you a fat-burner, and leave you feeling good, inside and out. I typically don't like to make hard-and-fast rules about what you can't eat; that said, it is helpful to know which foods will most sabotage your goals during the 4-Week Flexible Fasting Plan and beyond.

Sugar

Obviously, during your Clean Carb-Up days you can increase some of the whole-food-based or more natural sweeteners that I listed in that section. The following sweeteners are more processed and *should be avoided or significantly limited*. Make sure you read food labels carefully, because, as you learned earlier in this book, sugar is often disguised by another name. In fact, sugar can be hiding as any of the following on a food label.

- Agave nectar
- Agave syrup
- Barley malt
- Brown sugar
- Buttered sugar
- Cane juice crystals
- Cane sugar
- Caramel
- Castor sugar
- Confectioner's sugar
- Corn syrup
- Corn syrup solids
- Crystalline fructose
- Demerara sugar
- Dextrin
- Dextrose
- Diastatic malt
- Ethyl maltol
- Evaporated cane juice
- Florida Crystals
- Fructose
- Galactose
- Glucose (basically, anything with an -ose at the end is a no-go)
- Glucose syrup solids
- Golden sugar
- Golden syrup
- High-fructose corn syrup
- Icing sugar
- Invert sugar
- Lactose
- Maltodextrin
- Maltose
- Malt syrup
- Muscovado sugar
- Panela sugar
- Raw sugar
- Refiner's syrup
- Sorghum syrup
- Sucanat
- Sucrose
- Sugar (granulated or table)
- Turbinado sugar
- Yellow sugar

Artificial Sweeteners

Artificial sweeteners can be found in many diet and sugar-free drinks and foods, including the pervasive and endlessly popular diet sodas. Despite years of negative press surrounding sodas in general, one Gallup poll showed that the majority of adults still drink soda, and a large percentage choose "diet" versions—many probably believing their choice is healthier.[1] But is it? In my clinical opinion, no.

In fact, multiple studies have connected artificial sugars to autoimmune disease. For example, one case study from the American Association of Clinical Endocrinologists saw a complete reversal of autoimmune thyroiditis (Hashimoto's disease) in a patient by changing only one thing: eliminating artificial sweeteners and diet soda![2] Another study, published in the *World Journal of Gastroenterology,* correlated the rise of irritable bowel diseases, such as Crohn's disease and ulcerative colitis, with sucralose and its inhibitory effect on beneficial gut bacteria.[3] And finally, research published in the *Journal of Toxicology and Environmental Health* also points to sucralose's ability to weaken the microbiome.[4] The artificial sweetener was shown to reduce the good bacteria of the microbiome by up to 50 percent and also to raise gut pH levels. I believe it is plausible to theorize that this could trigger autoimmunity, considering that the microbiome is home to 80 percent of the body's immune system.

In addition, artificial sweeteners create confusion in your body and can sabotage your journey to metabolic flexibility, leading to cravings and weight loss resistance. That's why you'll want to avoid the following sweeteners during the 4-Week Flexible Fasting Plan and beyond:

- **Acesulfame**
- **Aspartame**—Equal, NutraSweet
- **Neotame**—a chemical derivative of aspartame found in various food products
- **Saccharin**—Sweet'N Low
- **Sucralose**—Splenda

Gluten-Containing Grains

Besides being high in carbs, most grains also contain gluten. In recent years, an explosion of gluten research has shed light on this troublesome protein, which is found in grains like wheat, rye, barley, spelt, and conventional oats. This protein is naturally occurring, but many people are sensitive to it, and it causes anything from digestive issues to leaky gut to autoimmune disease. In fact, one study linked gluten to fifty-five different chronic diseases.[5] Other research has shown that a piece of whole wheat bread can spike blood sugar just as much, if not more, than a can of soda.[6] Grains weren't always this way, but the hybridization of our grain supply to make it taste sweeter has created grains with "super" sugars and increased gluten content beyond what is naturally occurring, and both these concentrated sugars and elevated gluten can be disastrous to health.

It is my belief that everyone should get tested for gluten intolerance, if possible. That's because you don't necessarily have to be experiencing digestive problems to have an intolerance to gluten. In fact, many people have no idea just how much gluten is impacting their health. Even conservative estimates guess that one in twenty Americans has a gluten intolerance—which comes out to millions of people. Instead, look for grain-free options such as coconut flour, arrowroot starch, tapioca flour, plantain flour, and almond flour. Rice is one gluten-free grain that I find is generally more tolerated by people with gluten sensitivity. White rice is lower in lectin proteins and tends to be the most tolerable of the different rice varieties.

Unhealthy Fats

I know I've spent a lot of time convincing you that fat is healthy. But the truth is, it's a little more complicated than that. For a long time, there was an endless barrage of misinformation and propaganda against eating fat of all kinds. Now we know that not all fat is the same (in fact, there are four types of fat: monounsaturated fats, polyunsaturated fats, trans monounsaturated fats, and trans saturated fats). Some of these are healthy and some are unhealthy. And one of the best nutrition skills a person can have is the ability to distinguish between the two at a glance.

Here's what you need to know about the different types of fat.

Monounsaturated fats (MUFAs)

MUFAs include olive oil, avocado oil, and seed and nut oils, which are all liquid at room temperature but become solids when left in the fridge. MUFAs have been shown to support heart health and healthy cholesterol levels as well as to reduce the risk for stroke, diabetes, and visceral belly fat, which we know is the most damaging type of body fat. These fats are on the "healthy list."

Polyunsaturated fats (PUFAs)

PUFAs are the most confusing type of fats because some are healthy and some are not. PUFAs like those found in fatty fish, such as salmon and mackerel, and nuts and seeds, are good for you. The ones you want to avoid are the PUFAs found in foods like canola oil, soybean oils, safflower oils, and vegetable oils.

So what's the difference between the two types of PUFAs? The difference lies in the fact that some are naturally occurring and others are highly processed. Natural polyunsaturated oils can improve healthy cholesterol levels and calm inflammation. The processed, refined ones do the exact opposite, fueling inflammation and messing up your blood lipids. Avoid the refined kind—like those in canola oil, soybean oils, safflower oils, and vegetable oils—whenever possible.

Trans fats

This is the type of fat you've been warned about. Trans fats are created by altering the chemical makeup of natural fats by adding a hydrogen—hence the name "partially hydrogenated." This process increases the shelf life of the fat and makes it solid at room temperature, which makes it more convenient to use. That said, this hydrogenation also makes this fat incredibly dangerous; trans fats raise your LDL "bad" cholesterol and lower your HDL "good" cholesterol, which can lead to heart disease.

If you pick up most processed, packaged food in a grocery store and read the label, you will often see "partially hydrogenated oil" on it. These pesky fats are hiding in a ton of common foods—like creamers, spreads, and even cookies, cakes, and potato chips—where you wouldn't think to look for them. Trans fats are also commonly used in the fryers at restaurants and fast-food chains. As a general rule, do your absolute best to avoid this type of fat entirely.

Saturated fats (SFAs)

You may have already heard of saturated fats—like butter, ghee, coconut oil, eggs, and meats—probably in the context of heart disease. Well, if PUFAs win the award for the most confusing type of fat, SFAs are the most misunderstood. They have long been wrongly accused of being the primary cause of heart disease when, in fact, SFAs are necessary for healthy immune function, hormone health, cellular health, and feeding a healthy brain.

But what about heart disease? Well, the studies that saturated fat critics often cite to vilify these fats do not link eating more saturated fat to heart disease—rather, they link it to increasing cholesterol numbers. But the truth is that total cholesterol is a poor predictor for assessing heart attack and stroke risk. Studies have found that, in reality, there might be *no association* between high total cholesterol and heart attack and stroke risk.[7] In fact, a meta-analysis published in the *British Medical Journal* found no association between increased saturated fat intake and heart attack, stroke, and death risk.[8] A randomized controlled trial published in the *American Journal of Clinical Nutrition* found a diet rich in fats, including a high percentage of calories from saturated fats, actually lowered cardio-metabolic risk factors. More precisely, the results showed that HDL came up, triglycerides came down, insulin sensitivity improved, and blood sugar was lowered.[9]

The context and quality of a total cholesterol panel is so much more important than looking at a total cholesterol above 200 and deeming it "bad." Because it might not be bad at all. The research shows that saturated fats like coconut oil seem to improve the quality of cholesterol while also increasing the quantity. So what's a better predictor of heart attack and stroke risk? High inflammation markers, like C-reactive protein (CRP) and homocysteine, low HDL ("good" cholesterol), high triglycerides, and high small-density LDL protein particles.

The real problem with saturated fats like coconut oil occurs when people eat them with refined grains (which turn into sugar), such as breads and pasta or sugary foods. This "mixed meal" combination amplifies the inflammation of sugar. The good news is that during the 4-Week Flexible Fasting Plan, you're eliminating all refined grains and carbs anyway, so there's no need to worry about consuming moderate amounts of saturated fat during the plan.

There is one final exception to the saturated fats rule. Some people don't do well on saturated fats because of different SNPs (genetic variations) or underlying gut problems. For these people, focusing too much on saturated fats can increase inflammation. If you find that you don't do well eating higher amounts of saturated fats, try limiting saturated fat intake to 30 grams per day and, instead, focus on MUFAs and PUFAs.

Dairy

Dairy, like many foods, doesn't simply fall into a "good" or "bad" category. You probably grew up thinking that a glass of milk was the best way to start off your day, right? After all, it's filled with protein and calcium. After birth, we relied on fat in the form of breast milk for the first few months of our lives. The production of breast milk is a natural reaction in a mother's body because breast milk is exactly what a newborn needs to thrive outside of the womb. As we grow, that basic need for fat doesn't change.

So why isn't dairy recommended during the 4-Week Flexible Fasting Plan? Dairy is one of the most common allergens in our society. When you have a dairy intolerance, you are not able to break down the lactose—something called lactose intolerance. This occurs when the small intestine is not producing the enzyme lactase. While it is commonly thought that only a minority of the general public has this issue, the reality is that over 65 percent of the worldwide population, and up to 90 percent in some cultures, has an issue creating enough lactase.[10] And since this book focuses on healing the gut, reducing inflammation, and establishing metabolic flexibility, encouraging dairy just doesn't make sense.

This is not the only issue with dairy, though. Dairy also contains a protein called beta-casein, which has two subtypes, known as A1 and A2. Most conventionally run dairy farms in the United States use cows that have many gene mutations after thousands of years of crossbreeding, and they produce the A1 casein dairy that is sold in most grocery stores. This A1 casein is one of the main factors that increases inflammation in the body and can lead to digestive issues. On top of this, the cows producing this dairy are fed corn instead of grass, and their milk is pasteurized and homogenized, and the fat is removed. Many times, the dairy isn't the actual issue, it's what is done to the cows and the milk that makes it such an inflammatory food.

That is why other than grass-fed ghee (also known as clarified butter), we are avoiding dairy during the 4-Week Flexible Fasting Plan.

You're probably wondering why ghee is the exception. Well, grass-fed ghee is the only dairy that I'm encouraging during the fasting plan because it's a convenient and healthy alternative to butter, and it's great for cooking. First, the beta-casein is removed from ghee, which means all that's left is grass-fed clarified butterfat that contains fat-soluble vitamins—such as vitamins A, D, and K_2—that many of us are deficient in. Because ghee is a healthy fat source derived from animals, it also has a high smoke point. Most conventionally used oils have low oxidation levels and can form things like free radicals when heated. Ghee has a smoke point of 485 degrees Fahrenheit, so it's a great option to use when cooking and baking.

Ghee is also a decent source of medium-chain triglycerides, or MCTs, which make up about 25 percent of its fat content. MCT fats can help improve memory, increase muscle strength, and reduce toxin buildup. MCTs also enhance the effects of nutritional ketosis, which, in turn, encourage weight loss. In addition, the MCTs found in ghee can improve liver function, cholesterol, blood sugar, kidney function, and your immune system, and help you dive deeper into ketosis.

If you're a lover of all things cheese and dairy, don't worry. After the four weeks are over, you can add back in organic cheeses in moderation—as long as they don't upset your stomach.

Alcohol

We all know that chronic heavy alcohol use and its related disorders are bad for our health. When alcohol intake becomes severe, it can lead to an increased risk for liver disease, cancer, diabetes, neurological complications, bone damage, and many more inflammation-related conditions, according to the Mayo Clinic.[11] But the truth is, even moderate or mild alcohol intake can affect your health. For example, a report from the American Institute for Cancer Research showed that just one drink a day could increase a person's risk for breast cancer.[12] Another study, published in the *British Medical Journal,* showed that even moderate amounts of alcohol can affect your memory.[13] Often I see patients who do everything "right" but still have issues with their gut, mood, anxiety levels, and inflammation levels. And, often, eliminating those few drinks on the weekend or a glass of wine at night is the answer.

One big reason for this is the fact that alcohol immediately converts to sugar when it enters the body. If you truly want to invest in this plan and shift from being a sugar-burner to a fat-burner, cutting out alcohol is a must. The way I see it, there's no doubt that alcohol can be inflamma-tory, mostly because of the burden it puts on your GI tract and your liver, which houses your body's detoxification sys-tem. In addition, alcohol can affect your blood sugar, cause poor sleep, and lead you to indulge in processed and sugar-filled foods and abandon your "fasting window," which can sabotage the whole fasting plan.

Therefore—and while I hate to ruin the party—I recommend eliminating alcohol for the entirety of the 4-week fasting plan. The good news is that, according to a study from the University of Sussex, going a month without alcohol will benefit your health in more ways than one.[14] The study showed that those who participated in the "Dry January" alcohol challenge reported improvements in their health and their relationship with booze. More specifically, the results showed that:

- 71 percent slept better.
- 67 percent had more energy.
- 58 percent lost weight.
- 57 percent had better concentration.
- 54 percent had better skin.

When the four weeks of the plan are over, I recommend that you treat alcohol like sugar. In other words, it's a treat—which is meant to be consumed only occasionally and in true moderation. If you want to add some alcohol back in, you can. Just stick to clean, low-sugar alcohol like tequila, mescal, and organic dry red wine.

Mindful Eating and Overeating

You now have all the tools at your fin-gertips to make sure you're eating the healthiest foods possible to synergistically enhance your fasting plan. That said, I'd be remiss if I didn't talk about another crucial factor, which is how you actually consume your food.

You see, some research suggests that fasting can set some people up for over-eating when they break their fast. One study showed that going 24 hours with-out food was a strong predictor of future onset of recurrent binge eating.[15] This is definitely something we want to avoid and is exactly why I am not advocating that you try to intermittent-fast your way out of a poor diet. By pairing the ebbing and flowing fasting windows of your plan with a nutrient-dense, filling, and deli-cious fasting-mimicking Ketotarian diet, we are creating a sustainable lifestyle for you, not just another fad crash diet.

Part of creating a sustainable relation-ship with food is learning that it's not only what you put on your plate, but also the mind and heart space in which you eat that food—the art of mindful eating. The intention with which you eat your food is just as important as the food itself. In practice, that means sitting down to eat your meals without any distractions (that means no TV or phone!). Take a moment to smell your food, chew it fully, and don't rush. You might find that when you give your meal your full attention, it tastes way better and you naturally eat just until you're full—and not beyond that.

Mindfulness also applies to times when you're not eating. Maybe you're in your fasting window, but you're dying for a cookie. Or maybe you just ate your Break-a-Fast meal, but you're still feeling hungry. Whatever the situation, step back and take a few deep breaths, inhaling through your nose and exhaling through your mouth. Maybe make yourself a cup of tea and while you sip it, observe any thoughts and emotions that come up. Notice any urges you have to eat or indulge in certain foods.

And then, that's it! You don't have to do anything about those emotions or urges other than notice them with no judgment or resistance. This is how you grow your mindfulness muscle, which helps you get yourself back into the present moment and connect with your intuition. This is particularly important during the first couple of weeks of this plan, when your body is still struggling with metabolic inflexibility and you're just learning to reconnect with your intuition. Often you'll find that by just pausing for a second and noticing what's going on inside, your craving and hunger subside.

If they don't, that's okay, too. Remember, intermittent fasting is not about calorie restriction, and I want you to feel fully satisfied. If you still feel hungry after a meal or you're starving during your fasting window, go ahead and eat something that is high in clean protein and healthy fat, since those are the most satiating macronutrients. Don't beat yourself up about this. I've designed the plan in this book to be flexible—it's important that you embrace that part of the plan and be kind to yourself.

If you get through the plan and notice that you haven't felt the urge to overeat at all, this is also an outcome that is backed by science. For example, a large review of current research shows the opposite—that compared to other weight loss methods, fasting does not lead to overeating.[16] And as we have learned in the previous chapters, fasting can promote healthier hunger signals and more balanced blood sugar and can support a healthy gut and fewer cravings—all of which can greatly improve your ability to eat more mindfully and maintain healthy moderation when it comes to food.

Either way, the first rule of this book is to always listen to your body and take as much time as you need to gain metabolic flexibility, whether you're having a day filled with cravings or not. With intuitive fasting, our focus is never to push the body further than feels natural and doable. This book is more about filling your cart and your plate with clean, nutrient-dense foods—and then eating those foods mindfully and with gratitude—than it is about simply fasting for a certain number of hours.

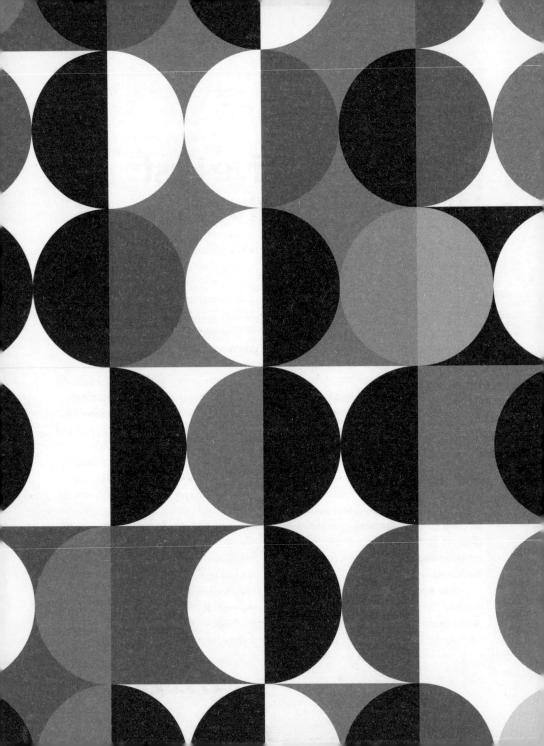

CHAPTER 10

Your Intuitive Fasting Toolbox

By now, I hope you've learned that the 4-Week Flexible Fasting Plan isn't just about fasting. In fact, nutrition plays an equally important role in the plan and its ability to restore your metabolic flexibility and enhance the benefits of your fasts. Well, the truth is, the plan doesn't end with nutrition recommendations, either.

If you want to establish metabolic flexibility, you have to be conscious of what you're eating, how you're eating, and when you're eating. That said, if you want to radically transform your health, you have to pay attention to all lifestyle factors, including non-food lifestyle factors like getting high-quality sleep, managing stress, moving your body, and making sure your body is getting all the vitamins and minerals it needs to function at optimal capacity and heal.

That's what this chapter is all about. Throughout the following sections, I'll give you all the tools you need to make

sure that you're getting the absolute most out of your 4-Week Flexible Fasting Plan.

How to Break a Fast: A Timeline

After a nice long period of time without food, what you supply your body as you transition out of a fast sends it a strong message. If you break your fast with a bunch of refined carbs and sugar, you'll spike your blood sugar, disrupt your gut, and serve as an unintentional saboteur to the progress you made over the course of the fast.

But if you break your fast gently, with a clean meal, you send your body the right signals, give it all the nutrients it *really* needs, and essentially supercharge the benefits of your fast.

Keep in mind that the longer the fast, the more important these recommendations are. If it's Week 1 or Week 4 and you've only fasted for 12 hours, you probably don't need to incorporate a transition meal. But if you've been fasting for 18 to 22 hours, I'd recommend easing your body back into its eating window as gently as possible and at least trying the full recommendations in this section to see how they positively impact your transition.

So without further ado, here's exactly how to ease your body into your daily eating window.

At the end of your fasting window, have a lighter Break-a-Fast meal that incorporates broth, soup, a smoothie, or soft, cooked food. My favorite options for this are bone broth, seaweed broth, or soups made from the broth. This will help support your gut's mucosal lining and your intestinal villi, which will help your body prepare to digest and absorb the food you eat.

- Organic bone broth: Loaded with minerals and electrolytes, this nutrient-dense, gut-soothing food is a great way to prep your gut to break your fast.

- Organic seaweed broth: A great plant-based option, seaweed broth contains beneficial minerals like selenium, zinc, and iodine, which will work together to support your thyroid and gear up your metabolism for your eating window.

Alternatively, on some days you could make a customized Ketotarian smoothie as your Break-a-Fast meal. For example: put almond or coconut milk, greens, some berries, and any superfood you like, such as spirulina, in a blender and blend with ice.

You can also eat soups or softer cooked foods that would be gentle on your digestive system, which could mean a roasted vegetable, cooked greens, and a gentle protein source like hard-boiled eggs. This meal should be smaller, lower in fat, lower in carbs, and have a moderate amount of protein. You should eat it slowly, making sure to chew your food completely before swallowing it. Avoid eating too many raw vegetables or fruits at this time, since these can be harder on your GI tract. Remember, your gut has been resting and repairing on your fast. Your goal with this meal should be to make it as simple and digestible as possible. The good news is that in chapter 13, there's a section featuring Break-a-Fast transition meal recipes.

After a longer fast, you will be extra insulin sensitive, your cortisol level will be higher, and your adrenaline level will be higher. All of this is normal and part of the beneficial hormetic effect I mentioned earlier. Because of this, I recommend adding some Himalayan pink sea salt and cinnamon into this meal in some way. These two ingredients will help stabilize blood sugar, keep you hydrated, and help your body ease into your eating window even more gently.

1 to 2 hours into your eating window—have a bigger meal. An hour or two after your transitional Break-a-Fast meal, you can eat your first real meal of the day. This meal can be larger and higher in fat since your body is now geared up to break down and digest a larger meal with a more complex mix of macronutrients. If you're on a Clean Carb-Up day, your main meal can also include your carbs for the day. You still want to make sure that this meal is a healthy one. That way, you know you're hitting the nail on the head and maximizing the benefits of the 4-Week Flexible Fasting Plan.

What to Consume During Your Fast

When I introduce my patients to intermittent fasting, the first questions they typically ask are: What is okay to consume during my fasting period? Is coffee okay? What about a latte? Bone broth? MCT oil?

What about supplements? In general, you want to try to avoid consuming anything with considerable calories during your fast. That means no snacks, no spoonfuls of nut butter, no juices or smoothies or soups or broths. Here are some good fasting liquids:

Water (and Lots of it)

Staying properly hydrated is, arguably, one of the most important things you can do for your overall health. Water not only prevents dehydration, it helps keep your body cool, keeps your skin supple, allows your body to flush out toxins, prevents issues like kidney stones and urinary tract infections, and prevents joint pain and muscle fatigue. Being properly hydrated has been associated with a better mood, fewer headaches, more energy, better brain function and concentration, less constipation, and even weight loss. Staying hydrated will support your body while it adjusts to burning fat for fuel and will ease the transition to metabolic flexibility.

That's why you should feel free to drink as much water as you want during your fasts and during your eating window. Exactly how much water depends on your activity level, how much you are sweating, and your age. Drink enough that you feel hydrated and not thirsty, and drink water throughout the day rather than all at once. If you are prone to waking up to urinate in the middle of the night, don't drink any water for a few hours before bedtime. If your urine is pale yellow and you feel good, then you are hitting your water target. You should start this hydration routine in Week 1 to prevent any unwanted side effects from fasting, such as constipation or headaches, and you should continue to maintain a healthy water intake throughout the 4-Week Flexible Fasting Plan. Water drinking tips:

1. Avoid drinking tons of water right before you eat, as it can interfere with digestion.

2. Drink your water at room temperature, or at least without ice, since cold water can be a shock to the body and cause stomach pains and cramps.

3. Water can even reduce hunger, so make sure you're drinking plenty of water during your fasts, especially if you're experiencing cravings or you're thinking about breaking your fast early.

When it comes to water, quantity isn't the only factor to consider. Quality matters, too. In 1974, Congress passed the Safe Drinking Water Act, which improved water quality nationwide, but we could still do better. This act regulates only 91 pollutants, and most drinking water contains many more contaminants that aren't regulated. One study found 316 contaminants in the U.S. drinking water, and a staggering 202 of those contaminants had no safety standards.[1] An estimated 132 million Americans in forty-five states have unregulated pollutants in their tap water! Also, a *New York Times* investigation estimated that over a five-year period, 62 million Americans were exposed to drinking water contaminated with thousands of unregulated chemicals.[2]

Pretty messed up, right?

This becomes even more worrisome when you learn that many of the contaminants found in our water have been linked to chronic health problems, including cancer, autoimmune-inflammation diseases, diabetes, thyroid problems, brain diseases, as well as liver, kidney, and nervous system problems. Even fluoride, which has been added to drinking water intentionally, could be linked to some serious health concerns. A scientific review of the Environmental Protection Agency's drinking water regulations suggested that tap water treated with fluoride was associated with increased rates of bone fractures and dental problems.[3] The study also recommended further investigation into fluoride's impact on thyroid and brain health.

This is why I not only recommend that you drink plenty of water during the 4-Week Flexible Fasting Plan but that you also invest in a water filtration system if at all possible, or at least purchase clean water. Do what you can. Here's what to look for:

There are many different brands of these filters on the market, and they are not all created equal. When buying your filter, look for these National Science Foundation (NSF) standards on the label:

- NSF Standard 42—Aesthetic Effects: This level of filtration reduces only chlorine and improves the taste and smell of your water.

- NSF Standard 53—Health Effects: This is the next level of filtration. Look for this standard to remove more chemicals and heavy metals.

- NSF Standard 58—Reverse Osmosis: This standard applies only to reverse osmosis systems and removes many toxic pollutants.

- NSF Standard 401—Emerging Compounds/Incidental Contaminants: This standard covers up to fifteen contaminants found in tap water, such as pharmaceutical drugs, heavy metals, and flame retardants.

Electrolytes

During all your fasts, but especially during your longer fasts, it's important to make sure you're staying properly hydrated, not just with water but also with electrolytes. Typically, water and fresh, hydrating fruits and veggies provide all the electrolytes you need. But when you're fasting, eating low-carb, and especially if you're exercising or live in a hot, humid climate, you may need to supplement with additional electrolytes. This is because you lose electrolytes through your sweat (in every liter of sweat, you lose 900 mg of sodium, 15 mg of potassium, and 13 mg of magnesium). Also, a low-carb diet cuts out inflammatory carbohydrates, which can result in water loss, throwing off your electrolyte balance.

Electrolytes is a word that gets thrown around a lot, but many of us aren't entirely clear as to what, exactly, they are. Electrolytes are compounds that produce positive or negative ions when they're dissolved in water. They just so happen to also play an important role in our health, regulating anything from nerve function to the fluid balance in our cells to blood pressure and the pH balance in our bodies. The major electrolytes are sodium, potassium, calcium, bicarbonate, magnesium, chloride, and phosphate, but there are also other trace minerals and elements that play a role in optimal hydration.

And before you pick up a bright blue bottle of *who-knows-what's-in-it* electrolyte drink, you should know that most electrolyte drinks are chock full of artificial or regular sugar, preservatives, and artificial colors and preservatives—ingredients we're most definitely avoiding during the

4-Week Flexible Fasting Plan and hopefully beyond.

Rest assured, there are easy, cheap, and simple ways to replenish your electrolytes without sports drinks.

- **Himalayan pink sea salt:** One easy way to replenish your electrolytes is simply by adding Himalayan pink sea salt to your water, because it is so mineral-rich. I often ask my patients with brain-adrenal axis issues, which can also deplete the body's electrolytes, to add 1 teaspoon of Himalayan sea salt to a glass of water in the morning or add it to their meals.

- **Broth:** You can also dissolve 1 to 2 vegetable or chicken bone broth bouillon cubes in a cup of water. Then, adding some of my favorite electrolyte-rich foods like mushrooms and spinach will provide you with potassium and magnesium, important minerals for hydration.

- **Electrolyte supplements:** There are some great electrolyte supplements on the market. Just make sure you take a look at the ingredient list and check for sugar or anything artificial.

MCTs

MCT stands for medium-chain triglyceride, a high-quality fat found naturally in foods. MCTs can help you deepen your ketosis because your body can quickly convert them into usable energy for your cells. In the modern Western diet, MCT fats are largely excluded. They are a type of healthy saturated fat that is very easy for your body to break down for fuel, unlike LCT (long-chain triglyceride) fats. MCT oils can be found in two forms: natural and synthetic. Natural MCTs are found in coconut oil, dairy fats like ghee, and palm kernel oil. Two of my favorite sources of MCTs are coconut oil and grass-fed ghee, but MCTs are only a percentage of the total amount of fat content:

Coconut oil: 60 percent MCT
Palm oil: 50 percent MCT
Ghee: 25 percent MCT

So why am I suggesting MCTs as an option during your fast? Because they have negligible calories and no sugar, they will have little impact on your fast. As an added bonus, MCTs have a plethora of their own health benefits and can even help supercharge the benefits of your fast. For example:

- MCTs support brain health and improve memory.[4] They have even shown promise for people with mild to moderate Alzheimer's disease.[5]

- MCTs can help you become a more efficient fat-burner and help you increase ketone production (even when your carb intake is higher).[6, 7, 8] Taking MCTs during your fasting plan will help you ease your body deeper into ketosis and help it burn fat for fuel.

- MCTs provide a very quick, easily absorbable, usable form of energy, so they are perfect if you feel run down or fatigued.

- MCTs have antibacterial, antiviral, and antifungal abilities and support a healthy gut microbiome.[9, 10]

- MCTs can improve ketosis, which means they can also help with fat burning and weight loss. Studies have shown that they can help you feel fuller, increase your metabolic rate, and decrease the conversion of excess carbohydrates to fats.[11, 12]

- Studies have shown that MCT oil, like intermittent fasting, can help you lose weight around your hips and waist, as well as visceral fat.

- Research has demonstrated that eating MCT-rich foods can increase your exercise performance and enable you to work out longer during high-intensity exercise.[13]

- I've written a lot about the importance of healthy fats in this book so far. Well, studies have shown that the effects of DHA and EPA omega fats were enhanced when they were combined with MCT oils.[14] Take advantage of that fat synergy by adding MCTs to the mix!

- MCTs have demonstrated the ability to increase insulin sensitivity to reduce blood sugar imbalances.[15]

- Your body's doing a lot of detoxing during the 4-Week Flexible Fasting Plan, and MCTs can help protect your liver and GI tract.[16]

- Fasting has shown beneficial effects on cholesterol levels and heart health, and MCTs have also been shown to lower cardio-metabolic risk factors and LDL/HDL ratios.

You can lean on MCTs at any point during the 4-Week Flexible Fasting Plan, but I'd suggest them particularly on longer fast days and your low-carb days, although they are not necessary. I'd also suggest taking them before a strenuous workout mixed with a shot of espresso, especially if it's a fasted workout, to help you increase athletic performance. Look for MCT oil that is extracted from coconut oil to get pure MCT fats and nothing else, or add a little coconut oil and ghee to your tea or coffee.

Before we move on, a word of advice: When it comes to MCTs, start off slowly. Too much can cause your stomach to cramp and lead to diarrhea. I recommend 1 teaspoon a day as a starting point, and you can work your way up to 2 to 3 tablespoons a day. You can incorporate MCTs during your fast by mixing them into coffee, tea, and water, and also during your eating window by mixing them into salad dressings, smoothies, bone broth, and soups.

Supplements and Medications

Before jumping into the 4-Week Flexible Fasting Plan itself, you should always talk to your doctor about how your medications and supplements fit into a fasting protocol. As a general rule, try to take any supplements and medications during your eating window since we are avoiding having to digest anything during our fasting window. This is particularly important for supplements that are gel capsules or contain calories (this will be listed on the nutritional label) or any sugar or flavoring.

The exception to this is, of course, if you've been instructed by your doctor or pharmacist to take your supplements or medications at a specific time of day. Some common medications that need to be taken at specific times of the day include:

- Antacid medications
- Antidepressants
- Bisphosphonates
- Blood pressure medications
- Diabetic medications
- Diuretics
- Migraine drugs
- Statin drugs
- Thyroid medications

These are just a few examples, so make sure you research any medications you're on to see if there are specific instructions

about what time of day they should be taken, and whether they should be taken with or without food. If there is a specific protocol, continue to take them at the prescribed time or talk to your doctor to see if there's any wiggle room. If you have to take a supplement or medication during your fast, it's not the end of the world. This is a *flexible* fasting plan! Don't stress about it, move on, and know that you're still getting the vast majority of the benefits.

Coffee

Coffee is a controversial topic in the wellness world. For the purposes of the 4-Week Flexible Fasting Plan, coffee consumption is allowed as long as you're not adding any milk or sugar. Why? Because coffee contains zero calories and zero sugar and may actually help you establish metabolic flexibility. Coffee has displayed inflammation-fighting, fat-burning, and insulin-balancing properties and is also a great source of antioxidants. There is also some evidence that coffee and caffeine can reduce appetite and even help your body burn more calories.

For coffee lovers, this is great news! Feel free to keep enjoying your coffee throughout the plan—there's no need to feel like you have to deprive yourself of your favorite drink! If you're used to coffee with milk and sugar and want a fasting-friendly creamy coffee recipe, try making your coffee keto-friendly by adding MCTs.

Fasting Coffee

MAKES ONE 8-OUNCE COFFEE

1 tablespoon grass-fed
  ghee

1 tablespoon coconut oil
  or MCT oil

1 cup freshly brewed,
  organic coffee

Using a blender or a hand-held milk frother, blend all ingredients until frothy.

By adding healthy fats to your coffee, you are giving your brain exactly what it needs to be mentally sharp and your body what it needs to be physically energized.

All that said, you don't want to overdo it, either. Coffee contains caffeine, which is a powerful drug. Drink too much and you can end up with anxiety, insomnia, digestive issues, heart palpitations, high blood pressure, panic attacks, nervousness, and even nausea and vomiting. You don't need me to tell you that these are things you want to avoid. My recommendation is to continue with your typical coffee habits throughout the plan. It's definitely not the time to increase your caffeine intake or start drinking caffeine for the first time.

This is particularly true if you think you might have a hormonal imbalance or a caffeine sensitivity. One gene variant, which codes for the enzyme CYP1A2, causes people to metabolize caffeine more slowly. I often test to see if my pa-

tients have this genetic variant because slow metabolizers don't do well with any caffeine; even a small cup will leave them feeling jittery and with a racing heart. If you think coffee might be an issue for you, the 4-Week Flexible Fasting Plan is a great opportunity to decrease your consumption and see how you feel.

Here's what I suggest:

Week 1: Cut your total daily coffee consumption by 25 percent, avoiding any caffeine after 5 p.m.

Week 2: Cut your total daily coffee consumption by 50 percent, avoiding any caffeine after 3 p.m.

Week 3: Cut your total daily coffee consumption by 75 percent, avoiding any caffeine after noon.

Week 4: Cut your total daily coffee consumption by 100 percent, avoiding any caffeine after noon.

So if you typically drink 2 coffees a day, during Week 1 reduce that to 1½ coffees a day. Then, in Week 2, reduce it to 1 coffee a day. In Week 3, make it half a cup a day, and in Week 4, don't have any coffee at all.

Tea

Tea is one of my absolute favorite wellness rituals, so I'm saving the best for last (in my humble opinion). As I have mentioned, tea is a great drink to have during your fasts . . . and, honestly, who am I kidding, anytime is a good time to drink tea!

Whether I am fasting or not, when I'm consulting patients via webcam at my functional medicine center, you will see me sipping on a variety of different tea elixirs. If you've never been much of a tea drinker, don't worry. On the following pages I'm going to show you everything you need to know about the wonderful world of tea, including which teas to drink to help supercharge the benefits of your 4-Week Flexible Fasting Plan. The world of tea truly offers something for everyone, depending on your taste, mood, and health goals.

First, let's test your tea trivia knowledge. Did you know that all true tea comes from the tea plant *Camellia sinensis*? That's right: black tea, green tea, white tea, and oolong tea all come from the same plant! What makes them so unique in look and taste is the way they are grown, harvested, and prepared. Even though teas tend to have less caffeine than most coffees,

all true teas have caffeine. All true teas also have antioxidant, antibacterial, anti-inflammatory, and antiviral benefits due to their antioxidant content, but what makes them different is their individual benefits, which can help you better decide which tea is best for you and your health.[17]

So without further ado, let's meet the family!

White Tea: The Virgin

This tea is made from the brand-new growth buds and young leaves of the tea plant. In order to inactivate oxidation, the leaves and buds are steamed and then dried. Since it is minimally processed, its antioxidant content is slightly higher than that of other varieties of tea.[18] It is characterized by its light color and mild flavor. It is an extremely easy tea to drink and has the lowest caffeine content of all tea types, making it a great choice if caffeine isn't your thing but you still want a little pick-me-up during your fast.

Green Tea: The Grounder

The Beyoncé of tea, green tea is definitely the most popular tea of the moment. While harvested later than white tea, green tea does not go through the same oxidation process that oolong and black tea go through. As with white tea, this allows for some of the highest levels of catechins, specifically the uber-beneficial compound epigallocatechin-3-gallate (EGCG). It's been shown in a number of exciting studies to be extremely powerful in a number of health issues.[19] It:

- Boosts metabolism
- Improves the skin
- Slows down aging
- Decreases cancer growth
- Improves brain function
- Protects from brain diseases
- Reduces heart disease risk
- Reverses diabetes
- Decreases inflammation

Thanks to these amazing properties, drinking green tea during a fast will only amplify the benefits of fasting itself. Like all the varieties of beer or wine, green tea comes in different forms that each have their own individual taste and array of nutrients and won't give you a hangover. Here's how the different green teas rank:

- **Matcha:** Matcha is a green powder made from a specific kind of green tea leaf. Unlike many other green teas, plants used for matcha are first covered and grown in the shade for weeks upon weeks before they are harvested, resulting in boosted chlorophyll levels, which gives the tea the bright green color it is known for. The leaves are then dried and ground into powder. Matcha has one of the highest concentrations of EGCG of all green teas, up to three times more than a typical sencha![20]

- **Sencha:** Sencha is brewed by infusing whole tea leaves in water to produce a very mild and pleasant taste. Harvested early on in the season, sencha is made from some of the most flavorful top leaves. It's no wonder that this is the most popular tea in Japan.

- **Gyokuro:** Gyokuro is similar to sencha, the biggest difference being that gyokuro, like matcha, is grown in the shade, giving it a milder flavor than sencha, which is grown in the sun and therefore has a stronger, more intense flavor. Gyokuro is also touted as having the highest EGCG levels.

- **Bancha:** More bitter in taste, bancha has the lowest caffeine content of all green tea varieties. It is harvested from the same tree as sencha, but later in the season, making it one of the cheapest, most commonly found green teas out there.

Oolong Tea: The Underdog

If black, green, and white tea are Destiny's Child, oolong is the overlooked member of the group who got kicked out sometime in the late '90s. But oolong is awesome! One of the biggest benefits of oolong tea comes from its weight-management properties. As with green tea, studies have shown that regularly drinking oolong tea can help prevent obesity by reducing weight through boosting fat metabolism, or lipolysis.[21] It can even suppress the creation of new fat cells![22] You therefore won't be surprised that I'd recommend drinking oolong throughout the 4-Week Flexible Fasting Plan if weight loss is one of your goals.

Black Tea: The Classic

When the tea leaf is harvested to make black tea, enzymes are activated, resulting in oxidation, leading to a withering of the leaves. Depending on the specific temperature and humidity controls, the leaves brown, and the desired taste and aroma are achieved. Many types of black tea are blends of different varieties of black tea from different regions. Black tea also has the highest caffeine content of all tea types. And since all black tea is oxidized, the catechins originally present are converted to theaflavins. While the high catechin content in green tea is a major health benefit, studies have shown that theaflavins are just as powerful antioxidants, making black tea a perfect choice if you need a boost of caffeine but still want the antioxidant power.[23] Black tea don't tend to differ too much in health benefits; choosing the right one for you is really a matter of taste.

- **English Breakfast Tea:** One of the most popular types of black tea is English breakfast tea. A blend of Assam, Kenyan, and Ceylon varieties of black tea, to everyone in the United Kingdom, this is the only tea that exists.

- **Earl Grey Tea:** Good ol' Earl. Earl Grey tea is a black tea that traditionally

includes bergamot oil. Beyond taste, I love Earl Grey for its health benefits. Earlier in this book, we learned about autophagy; well, bergamot can actually help enhance and support autophagy. In fact, bergamot oil is one of the polyphenols that contain natural healing properties at cellular levels that increase and induce the autophagy process.[24] These polyphenols are compounds found in plants that protect the plant from any damage. And as bergamot oil protects the plant, when eaten it also protects our bodies by boosting our autophagy process. Including bergamot in your fasting plan will help support your body's ability to clean out damaged cells as well as promote new cell growth. Personally, I sip on organic Earl Grey tea to enhance autophagy when I am doing intermittent fasting—and I make sure it has real bergamot, not just bergamot flavoring. If you don't have Earl Grey tea on hand, you can mix a drop or two of pure bergamot essential oil into black tea to create the same taste and benefits of Earl Grey. Bergamot oil can also be added to different kinds of food, like dips and desserts, to given them a hint of citrus flavor.

- If you're not a Fasting Coffee drinker (see recipe on page 133) or just want to take an Earl Grey latte for a spin to spice up your caffeine intake during your fasting window, try this keto-friendly take on a traditional London fog recipe:

Fasting London Fog

1 Earl Grey tea bag
1 cup hot water
¼ tsp vanilla extract
1 tablespoon grass-fed ghee
1 tablespoon coconut oil or MCT oil
Keto sweetener to taste

Brew tea in hot water—covered—for 3 to 5 minutes. Then, using a blender or a hand-held milk frother, blend all ingredients together until frothy.

A note on shopping for tea: Contamination is an issue for many tea brands, so I recommend always looking for organic tea whenever possible. Heavy metals such as lead can be found in many plant products, because it is absorbed from the soil, and tea is known to absorb lead at a higher rate. White tea, because it is picked sooner, is known to have lower amounts on average. An easy solution, if you don't want to just drink white? Avoid non-organic tea from China. Studies have found that Chinese industrial pollution causes the leaves to have higher lead levels.[25] I suggest getting your tea only from Japan, where contamination is less of a problem.

Herbal Tea

If caffeine isn't your jam or you just want more variety, herbal teas are made from a combination of single herbs, plants, fruits, and spices and differ from the aforementioned varieties by the fact that they contain zero caffeine. But what they lack in caffeine they make up for in their incredible and diverse health benefits. Chances are, whatever health problem you are dealing with, there is an herbal tea to help remedy your symptoms. There are many more types of herbal tea than just the ones on the following list, but if I included all of them, they would fill this entire book! Instead, let this be your go-to tea guide for the most common health problems I see among my patients. So grab your favorite mug and start steeping away your health woes one cup at a time.

ANXIETY AND STRESS

- **Chamomile:** Chamomile promotes relaxation and has been shown to decrease symptoms of anxiety.[26]

- **Kava:** This herb is one of the common natural anti-anxiety treatments out there.[27]

- **Passionflower:** Studies have concluded that this herb can be just as effective as the tranquilizer oxazepam in treating anxiety because of its assumed GABA-increasing abilities, which promote relaxation.[28]
- **Tulsi:** This herb has been used in Ayurvedic medicine for a long time, and it also goes by the name Holy Basil. Tulsi acts as an adaptogen, supporting a balanced HPA axis (hypothalamic-pituitary-adrenal axis, or brain-adrenal axis)—that is, your body's stress response.

BEAUTY

- **Rooibos:** This South African tea is loaded with antioxidants to help fight against the free radical damage responsible for skin aging.
- **Rosehip tea:** This tea not only also fights against free radical damage but increases cell rejuvenation to keep skin youthful longer.

BLOOD SUGAR BALANCE

- **Bilberry:** The powerful flavonoids known as anthocyanosides have shown promising results in maintaining blood sugar balance.[29]
- **Hibiscus:** Research has shown that hibiscus can help inhibit the absorption of glucose in the body and therefore keep blood sugar more balanced.[30]

- **Lemon balm:** Lemon balm replenishes the nervous system and helps regulate insulin production.

DETOXIFICATION

- **Burdock root:** A natural diuretic, this tea can help remove excess toxins, particularly heavy metals, through increased fluid excretion. It can also boost your lymphatic system and allow for increased detoxification.
- **Dandelion:** Dandelion has powerful liver-supporting properties to help flush out toxins from the body.
- **Red clover:** Red clover aids in cleansing the liver, lymphatic system, and spleen of toxins.

FATIGUE

- **Licorice:** Licorice balances out uneven cortisol levels.[31]
- **Rooibos:** African red bush tea can have a balancing effect on your body's main stress hormone, cortisol.[32]

GUT HEALTH

- **Licorice:** Deglycyrrhizinated licorice (DGL) helps heal and repair damaged gut lining.
- **Peppermint:** Studies have shown that this herb is able to bring relief to those suffering from irritable bowel syndrome (IBS) by helping reduce inflammation.[33]

- **Marshmallow root:** No, not your sugar-filled camping dessert, this root actually helps repair damaged gut lining in order to treat leaky gut syndrome. It also helps coat the stomach and ease symptoms of heartburn, constipation, and diarrhea.

- **Slippery elm:** This specific variety of elm tree is a known demulcent able to reduce inflammation of the digestive system to relieve symptoms of IBS, leaky gut syndrome, and other gut problems.

IMMUNITY

- **Echinacea:** With its antibacterial and antiviral properties, there's a reason this herb is also found in the cold-and-flu aisle of your pharmacy.

- **Elderberry:** Hippocrates, the father of modern medicine, once referred to the elder tree as his "medicine chest" because of its extremely powerful anti-microbial and antiviral abilities, specifically against the flu.[34]

- **Hibiscus:** Because of its rich vitamin C content, hibiscus is a fantastic immune booster and can help when you feel a cold coming on.

INFLAMMATION

- **Nettle leaf:** Nettle is essentially an Nfkb inhibitor. Nfkb is a type of inflammation, and nettle helps quell it in your body.[35]

- **Ginger:** Often used to calm upset stomachs, ginger also brings down pro-inflammatory Nfkb activity and inhibits pro-inflammatory cytokines such as IL-1 and IL-8.[36]

- **Rose hips:** Since they contain a type of anti-inflammatory galactolipid, rose hips are able to aid in reducing symptoms of inflammatory conditions such as rheumatoid arthritis and IBS.[37]

Remember when we talked about the many underlying health imbalances that contribute to metabolic inflexibility and get in the way of your intuition about food? Well, tea can be a big part of healing those imbalances and getting back in touch with your body. And the best part is, you can take advantage of those benefits in the form of a tasty, zero-sugar beverage *during your fasting window*. I would definitely recommend picking a few teas to sip on during your 4-Week Flexible Fasting Plan.

Metaphysical Meals

Before we move on to the next section about sleep, another question I frequently get from my patients is: What do I do during mealtimes when I am fasting? At first, you may feel like your day has giant gaps in it, especially if you're skipping breakfast. This is normal. You've most likely woken up every morning for years thinking about what you're going to have for breakfast; now, you've taken that schedule and flipped it on its head. It's normal to feel a little lost and aimless when you're not spending your morning preparing breakfast, sitting down and eating, and then cleaning up. What should you do with all this extra time? I would argue that many times, the ritual of breakfast has less to do with the actual food than you think. In fact, I would argue that regardless of the meal that you're eliminating. I'd encourage you to fill the gap in your day with something mindful, such as a 10-minute meditation or prayer, a walk around the neighborhood or in nature, doing something creative, or doing some journaling. These are all examples of practices that I like to call Metaphysical Meals. With these rituals, you can still nourish yourself, even if it's not with food. As we already learned, cultures across the globe have used fasting as a spiritual tool for centuries. I'd encourage you to not spend your would-be mealtimes on television or social media and instead take that gift of a little extra time and spend it reflecting, slowing down, and getting to know yourself a little better. Use this time of stillness to look inward. The magic often hides in the spaces we are ignoring.

If you're not sure where to start, try some of these Metaphysical Meal journal prompts:

1. Make a list of ten things you're grateful for.

2. Make a list of things that make you feel nourished that have nothing to do with food.

3. Make a list of ten things you're looking forward to (get as specific as possible).

4. Make a list of things you want to let go of in your life.

5. Make a list of something you want to manifest in your life.

You can use the above journal ideas as meditation or prayer tools during your Metaphysical Mealtime. I love to use my time drinking tea to meditate.

This Metaphysical Mealtime is a great opportunity to reflect on healing your relationship with food and your body. If that's a relationship you'd like to explore, try these prompts:

1. Write down what food peace means to you.

2. Write down the patterns you've noticed when it comes to your emotional health and food.

3. Write down a list of adjectives you associate with food, fasting, and mealtimes.

As a functional medicine practitioner, I know that while intermittent fasting and proper nutrition are the backbones of metabolic flexibility, other factors like stress, sleep, and exercise can make the difference between your living your healthiest life, or not.

Sleep and Metabolic Flexibility

Many people think of eight hours of high-quality sleep as a luxury and that they will "sleep when they're dead." Sleep is not a luxury, it is a mandate on your health and metabolic flexibility. Why? Sleep is intricately connected to all the hormonal and metabolic processes in our bodies as well as to maintaining healthy inflammation levels, healthy blood sugar, and a healthy weight. Don't believe me? Studies have shown that just one night—yes, *one single night*—of sleep deprivation changes the way our hunger and appetite hormones behave, which leads to increased hunger and cravings.[38] One night of bad sleep can also affect the motivation centers in your brain and how they respond to the sight or thought of food. If you've ever pulled an all-nighter—only to be constantly hungry and craving bagels and potato chips and cookies the next day—you've experienced this phenomenon in action. Conversely, scientists have found that the more sleep you get, the less hungry you are and the less you crave sweet and salty foods.[39] If you don't get enough sleep, it's almost impossible to overcome cravings and wonky hunger signals in order to reconnect with your intuition about food and what your body really needs.

Studies have also shown that insulin sensitivity is negatively impacted by sleep deprivation.[40] In fact, one study showed that six nights of just four hours of sleep resulted in a 40 percent reduction in glucose tolerance.[41] Sleep deprivation also stimulates your sympathetic nervous system, your fight-or-flight nervous system.[42] This leads to increased stress hormones, and, as we already know, these can negatively affect our metabolism. Finally, poor sleep habits also lead to increased inflammation levels. For example, studies experimenting with sleep deprivation have revealed that it can alter the immune system's response and increase pro-inflammatory markers like IL-6, TNF-alpha, and C-reactive protein.[43, 44] In other words: sleep is pretty freaking important; in fact, I'd go as far as to say that if you're not prioritizing sleep, it's impossible to be truly healthy.

Prioritizing sleep is made even more complicated by the fact that getting great sleep is easier said than done. It's not as easy as other lifestyle factors like exercise or nutrition, where you simply have to do and eat the right things. According to the National Sleep Foundation, 35 percent of Americans consider their sleep quality "poor" or "only fair," and another survey showed that 68 percent of Americans struggle with sleep at least once a week.[45, 46]

So, how do we get great sleep? I work with my patients all the time to optimize their sleep, and I've found that the key is to establish a bedtime routine that sets you up to fall asleep quickly and easily—and then stay asleep all night long. Your routine can include anything that feels right to you: a bath, writing tomorrow's to-do list, a short meditation, or even just sitting in bed and reading. That said, there are a few elements you'll want to make sure you include:

- **Turn off all electronics an hour before bed:** This means smartphones, computers, and tablets. These devices emit blue light, which actually makes you feel more awake and reduces melatonin production, which is supposed to surge before bed. If you can't make it an entire 60 minutes before bed, aim for at least 30 minutes. Try reading, journaling, listening to an audiobook, or doing a few minutes of yoga instead.

- **No coffee after lunch:** Too much coffee throughout the day can interfere with our sleep. That's why I recommend avoiding coffee after lunch. This gives your system enough time to metabolize it fully before you hit the hay. Instead of coffee, try herbal tea, sparkling water, or a turmeric latte.

- **Go for a walk:** I know I've told you to avoid over-exercising during the 4-Week Fasting Plan, but moving your body in some way each day, even if it's just a 15-minute walk, can benefit your sleep massively. In fact, a study from the *Sleep Health Journal* showed that

daily active minutes could be directly linked to sleep quality.[47]

If you cut out electronic use before bed and caffeine in the afternoon and are still having trouble getting your daily dose of zzz's, it's time to lean on natural remedies like herbs and supplements. These are my go-to herbs and supplements for sleep:

- **Chamomile:** Chamomile is one of the most famous herbs around. It's been historically suggested for anything from sleeplessness and anxiety to gastrointestinal conditions such as upset stomach, gas, and diarrhea. More recent studies have shown that it can improve sleep measures in adults with chronic insomnia.[48] I recommend taking chamomile in tea-form after dinner.

- **Magnesium:** Magnesium is known as nature's chill pill. Magnesium can be very effective as a sleep aid, thanks to its ability to encourage muscle relaxation and improve measures of insomnia, as listed in the ISI (insomnia severity index), including sleep efficiency; sleep time and sleep onset latency; early morning awakening; and the concentration of serum renin, melatonin, and serum cortisol.[49] Studies have even shown that magnesium can regulate your sleep-wake cycle.[50] There is no "right" time to take magnesium. However, due to its calming effects, taking it right before bed can be the best way to capitalize on its ability to boost GABA levels and relax muscles. Magnesium can be found in multiple different forms, and I recommend starting with 200 mg after dinner.

- **Valerian:** Valerian is an herb that has been used to treat nervousness, trembling, headaches, insomnia, and heart palpitations since ancient Greece and Rome.[51] I recommend taking valerian as a tea after dinner.

- **L-theanine:** L-theanine is another go-to natural supplement for sleep. This compound is found naturally in green tea and, when taken as a supplement, can promote better sleep quality.[52] In fact, one study found that when boys ages 8 through 12 took L-theanine (at a dose of 400 mg daily), it led to improved sleep quality without any safety concerns.[53] I recommend that my patients start with 100 mg, but healthy adults can take up to 400 mg.

- **Melatonin:** We've already learned about the importance of melatonin for healthy sleep. But did you know that you can take melatonin as a supplement? It's true. If none of the strategies above are quite doing the trick—and you find yourself wide awake when you should be falling asleep—supplementing with melatonin can help. Melatonin has been widely studied for insomnia, especially insomnia related to jet lag, and the science is promising. One review paper showed that, in nine out of the ten studies they

evaluated, taking melatonin close to bedtime at the destination (between 10 p.m. and midnight) decreased jet lag from flights crossing time zones.[54] If you're having trouble sleeping during the 4-Week Flexible Fasting Plan, try taking 5 mg of melatonin about 30 minutes before you're ready to go to sleep.

Next, we're going to turn our attention to the opposite of sleep: exercise. When I suggest fasting to my patients, they often ask me how exercise fits into the plan. The 4-Week Flexible Fasting Plan is a great opportunity to start moving your body, too, but there's so much more to learn about how exercise fits into an intermittent fasting lifestyle. Keep reading for everything you need to know.

Exercise and Intermittent Fasting

Whenever I write, speak, or talk to my patients about intermittent fasting, I always get questions about exercise. How does exercise fit into a fasting plan? Should I exercise before, during, or after my fast? Should I be exercising at all?

Unfortunately, there's no cut-and-dried answer for how much a person should exercise during the four weeks. The answer depends on your typical activity level before the plan, how metabolically inflexible you are at the start, what your underlying health imbalances might be, and whether or not you experience any symptoms of keto flu or exhaustion throughout the four weeks. In this section, I'm going to give you the information you need to decide how much exercise is right for you during the 4-Week Flexible Fasting Plan.

First things first: This is not the time to start training for a marathon or to try CrossFit for the first time. Many of my patients are tempted to start doing everything at once during the 4-Week Flexible Fasting Plan, but if you overdo it, you'll just end up starving, sore, and exhausted. As a general rule, plan to *maintain your current level of physical activity,* and be prepared to pull back on the intensity or duration as needed. Always listen to your body. On some days you'll be brimming with energy and may even experience some of the best workouts of your life; other days, your energy level might be low as your body adjusts to leaning on alternative fuel sources, and you might feel lethargic from the start of your workouts or hit a wall halfway through. If this happens to you, don't push it and don't beat yourself up. You're making massive metabolic shifts right now—give your body the time and space it needs to establish metabolic flexibility.

Once you've cycled through all four weeks of the plan, you can step up your workouts and you'll likely feel roaring and ready to hit the treadmill, field, court, and weight room. But for now, don't stress too much about how intensely you're moving your body—just make sure you're getting your steps or maintaining your current level of exercise.

Fasted versus Non-Fasted Workouts

So now on to more logistical questions: When should you work out? Is it better to work out on an empty stomach before your fast ends or during your eating window? Unfortunately, the answer to this isn't as simple as we'd hoped for, either. The good news is that there are benefits to both fasted and non-fasted workouts.

When you're fasting, you don't have blood glucose to call upon for energy, and your stored form of carbohydrates—known as glycogen—are most likely depleted, which means your body will burn more fat, especially if you do cardio.[55] One study in particular demonstrates the benefits of fasted workouts.[56] Researchers divided 50 active, healthy men into three groups—one that didn't exercise at all; another that exercised after a high-carb breakfast and drank sports drinks during their workouts; and a third that drank only water and had their first meal after their workouts. The researchers had all three groups increase their calories and fat intake. The results showed that the men in the first and second groups gained weight and also showed unhealthy metabolic signs like insulin resistance. The third group, the fasted workout group, however, gained almost no weight and didn't show any signs of insulin resistance. In fact, the results showed that they actually burned off the extra fat they were consuming more efficiently. As an added bonus, working out on an empty stomach also simplifies your morning and prevents potential indigestion, which you can get from eating and then trying to do something intense while your body is digesting.

Here are some fasted workout tips to keep in mind:

- Start with low-intensity cardio exercise: I recommend light jogging, walking, or cycling.

- Slowly increase the intensity of your fasted workouts as your body adjusts.

- Save your harder workouts for your shorter fasting window days and your Clean Carb-Up days. That way, you can run, lift weights, go on a really long walk, or do whatever your version of high-intensity exercise is and then eat your carbs after. Exercise will make you more insulin sensitive and leptin sensitive and deplete your glycogen completely, which means your body is perfectly primed to burn those carbs instead of storing them as fat.

- Try to work out right before you break your fasts so you can replenish your body with healthy fats, proteins, vegetables, and carbohydrates while your metabolism is still revved up from the workout.

- Observe your energy levels closely to make sure your performance isn't suffering.

At first, you might be low-energy and feel a little wonky (yes, that's a technical term). This is because you're not only burning fat to fuel your brain and basic biological functions, you're requiring your muscles to learn to use less stored glucose and to use fat for fuel instead. Once you're more adapted to this new way of exercising, you might actually feel like you have more energy when you work out in a fasted state or notice that your body feels lighter and more agile.

All that said, these studies aren't the end-all, be-all. In fact, there are also studies that question whether you do actually burn more fat when you work out on an empty stomach.[57] Not to mention, you may hit a wall in the middle of your fasted workout or notice that you just can't train quite as hard when you're relying on fat for fuel. This is likely because glycogen, which is the stored form of glucose in the body, will be depleted after weeks of low-carb eating and fasting. Glycogen depletion can also upset hormones like progesterone, thyroid hormone, and leptin. This is why I don't recommend that you do all your workouts in the fasted state. It's great to mix it up; that way, you can get in some nice fat-burning cardio in a fasted state and maybe save your weight lifting or toning exercises for your eating window. That way, you'll have glycogen stored in your muscles and liver that is readily available and can be mobilized quickly to push you through a wall.

Mindful Movement

One of the biggest mistakes I see people make when it comes to moving their bodies is limiting what they consider to be a true "workout." Sure, "working out" can mean a 45-minute HIIT (high-intensity interval training) workout with burpees, squats, and star jumps galore—but it doesn't have to. We have to expand our view of workouts to include anything that gets our body moving for any amount of time. Let me say it louder for people in the back: *Anything that gets your body moving for any period of time is a workout*—and that means dancing to your favorite song, taking the stairs instead of the elevator, and even walking around the mall for the day. It also means tennis, gardening, or playing basketball with your kid. We often overvalue "workouts." What are you doing the other twenty-three hours a day? Make movement a lifestyle.

If you're new to exercise or don't have a sport or activity that you love, consider making a commitment to walking. Walking is simple: you don't need any fancy workout gear or a gym membership, and most of the time you don't even have to change your clothes before or after. You can walk on the sidewalk, in your back-

yard, or through your neighborhood. Many people raise their noses at the benefits of walking, but I'd argue that it might be the healthiest form of exercise. In fact, just like other forms of exercise, walking has been shown to improve cardiovascular risk factors such as high cholesterol, blood pressure, diabetes, obesity, vascular stiffness and inflammation, and mental stress. Not to mention, it will also protect against dementia, peripheral artery disease, obesity, diabetes, depression, colon cancer, and even erectile dysfunction.[58]

The people who live the longest don't have Equinox gyms and fancy Apple Watches to track their workouts. Instead, they garden, carry their groceries up the hill, and they walk—everywhere. In fact, in Old Order Amish communities, the average woman logs about 14,000 steps per day; these communities also have some of the lowest rates of obesity anywhere in America.[59]

This is no coincidence. The benefits of walking are impossible to argue with. For example, a study on 12,000 adults revealed that people who live in cities have a far lower risk of being overweight and obese than people who live in the suburbs.[60] For example, in the city of Atlanta, 45 percent of the men who lived in the suburbs were overweight compared with only 37 percent of men who lived in the city. The reason for this? You guessed it: city dwellers walk instead of drive.

I write all that to communicate that

expanding your perspective on what it means to move your body is critical during the 4-Week Flexible Fasting Plan, because, most likely, on some days you won't feel like you're up for a traditional 45-minute or hour-long workout. This is fine, but it doesn't mean you should sit on the couch all day, either. Instead, try a 20-minute walk, a 10-minute jog, or 5 minutes of stretching before bed. These small spurts of movement will help your body establish metabolic flexibility, keep your metabolism and muscles active throughout the day, fend off stress, and help you sleep more soundly, which, as we already know, are keys to your success.

I recommend moving your body to support overall health, but also as a go-to acute remedy if you're thinking about breaking your fast early. If you're feeling hungry, experiencing cravings, or you're experiencing any symptoms of keto flu, try moving your body for 5 minutes and notice how you feel. Most likely, it will get you out of your head and help you feel less stagnant, and you'll be able to continue with your fast.

How to Decrease Stress to Optimize Metabolic Flexibility

Hopefully, by now you see that it's not just about what you feed your body, but about what you feed your mind and soul, too. Stress can sabotage your endocrine system, raise your blood sugar, ruin your sleep, destroy your metabolic flexibility, and make you feel disconnected from your intuition. Stress is one of the hidden reasons why some people have a difficult time getting into ketosis, and stress is associated with endless health conditions. In fact, research suggests that about 90 percent of doctor visits are for stress-related illnesses, which include anything from heart disease, headaches, and anxiety to diabetes, asthma, and depression.

Unfortunately, many of us don't feel like we're able to effectively manage the stress we experience, and this is also an issue during the 4-Week Flexible Fasting Plan. Long-term low-carb diets can put additional stress on the adrenals, which can exacerbate an adrenal issue and cause uncomfortable symptoms like fatigue, insomnia, and anxiety. In fact, in my functional medicine practice, I discourage my patients from going low-carb long-term until they've addressed their unhealthy stress levels.

That's the bad news. The good news is that if you've already started to optimize your sleep and started moving your body, you've taken two giant leaps forward toward effective stress management. Sleeping well and exercising are absolutely key pieces of the stress management puzzle. In addition, if you're struggling with chronic stress, you'll definitely want to experiment with carb cycling, because, as we learned, you need some carbohydrates to effectively manage stress.

Clean Carb Cycling, sleeping well, and moving your body are no doubt crucial pieces of the stress management puzzle, but there are other strategies you can also implement to make sure your days are manageable. If you know that stress is a problem for you, you're not alone. I still struggle to manage stress in my own life at times. After years of practicing mindfulness, I've found that these are the practices that have helped me and my patients start managing stress and maximizing physical and mental health:

Have a Morning

Instead of hitting the snooze button one too many times, give yourself plenty of time to slowly wake up and start your day off on the right foot. Take the time to sip your morning beverage—whether it be coffee, tea, or just a glass of water—in silence, centering yourself for the day. Running around the house at the last minute starts your day off on a frantic, frazzled note.

Write a (Reasonable) To-Do List

And when I say reasonable, I mean reasonable. If you expect too much from yourself every single day, you'll always feel like you're behind, and that will cause a lot of undue stress. This will require you to weed out tasks that are not absolutely a priority that day. I recommend writing your to-do list in the morning, when you have a few minutes to reflect on your priorities for the day. Start with more pressing needs and work your way to longer-term goals. Then relish in the feeling of crossing things off that list as the day goes on. This approach will gather the mental clutter and organize it all into an orderly list. But also remember, if it all doesn't get done today, give yourself grace—there is always tomorrow.

Don't Try to Do Two Things at Once

As you are moving through the day's to-do list, try to dive as deeply as you can into the task at hand. Preoccupied thoughts about the future or the past can cause anxiety and decrease your effectiveness, causing a lot of stress. This is true even if the task at hand is boring, frustrating, or tedious. Don't just watch the clock tick by; however mundane your to-do may be, honor it. Fully accepting the task at hand decreases stress and can help bring you inner peace.

Get in Touch with Nature

Nature has been scientifically proven to put our minds at ease and increase our quality of life.[61] Studies have shown that people who spend time in green space are 50 percent less likely to report stress and that people living more than 1 kilometer away from green space are 50 percent more likely to experience stress than those living just 300 meters away.[62] The research coming out of South Korea and Japan on nature therapy is quite compelling. The Japanese term is *shinrin-yoku*. *Shinrin* in Japanese means "forest," and *yoku* means "bath." I recommend spending some amount of time in nature every single day if possible. Forest-bathe as much as you can. That could even mean a walk in the nearest park, lying outside in the grass, or taking a walk on the weekend.

Declutter Your Space

Decluttering your space can transform your mental state. Clutter on the outside can cause clutter on the inside, so take time each week to clean up your home, office, or workspace. Throw away anything that doesn't have a positive or practical purpose. Decluttering can also be a great remedy for tackling cravings during the 4-Week Flexible Fasting Plan. Feeling overwhelmed today and like you want to eat an entire bag of movie theater popcorn? Take five to ten minutes to organize your space and notice how it brings you peace of mind—and relief from your cravings.

Set Boundaries with Social Media

Speaking of decluttering your life, the 4-Week Flexible Fasting Plan is an excellent opportunity to turn your attention away from your devices and social media. If you're being bombarded with any content that makes your adrenaline rise or makes you feel like you should be doing more, be merciless about getting that content out of your zone. FOMO-inducing, stress-increasing endless scrolling of content online is detrimental to your health. Sometimes self-care means hitting the mute, unfollow, or turn-off-notifications buttons with abandon. Consider doing intermittent phone fasts. You can also set time boundaries with social media; for example, don't scroll before noon or after 8 p.m., saving your sharing and liking for the middle of the day. If you're not sure about this in the long term, commit to doing it for the 4-Week Flexible Fasting Plan and see how you feel by the end; I guarantee you'll feel more present, happier, and more content with your life when you're not spending quite so much time each day on everyone else's.

If you can set boundaries, get your home and office in order, and find time to be mindful in the morning, you may notice that your chronic daily stress melts away. That said, we all have those days when we just can't deal. For those moments, I recommend the breathing exercise at the end of this chapter. It's been studied extensively to help with acute stress.

How to Cultivate a Fasting-Friendly Community

In this chapter we're focusing on all the non-fasting, non-food-related things we can do to optimize the 4-Week Flexible Fasting Plan. And one of the big pieces of the puzzle is creating a supportive community that makes it easier for you to stay motivated.

Some of you will already be blessed with a supportive circle of friends and family members who bolster your efforts to establish metabolic flexibility and take fasting for a spin. Heck, they might even offer to do it with you! Some people feel much more motivated when they're part of a group; if you're one of those people, share this book with others and do it together.

That said, before you decide to get your friends involved, take a minute to think about whether they will really help your mission. We all have different personalities, and some people are better at doing things like this on their own.

Whether you're going through the plan solo or with a big group, you may feel like you're alone in this. At the end of the day, even if you have company, changing your diet and lifestyle can be an isolating thing. It's even possible that you'll receive some

judgment or criticism from those around you. If you suspect this may happen to you, remember this: just because something is common doesn't make it normal. Feeling lousy and eating unhealthy food is a really hot-button topic for people, and you may ruffle some feathers by changing things up. My advice is to write down, on paper, why you decided to take this journey and then read that note to yourself anytime someone makes you question your efforts.

If you're worried about how this plan, or fasting in general, will affect your social life, I hear you. So much of our social lives are centered around eating out—most of the time meals that involve a lot of bread and dessert—and drinking alcohol, both of which are absent from your 4-Week Flexible Fasting Plan. But that doesn't mean you need to hole up and become a recluse for four weeks; in fact, I strongly discourage staying home for a month. We should not feel like having a social life and living a healthy lifestyle are mutually exclusive—that's dangerous thinking! Instead, find fasting-friendly ways to socialize with friends. Here are some ideas to get you started:

- Go on a walk or do a workout with your bestie or your partner.
- Schedule your social time on Clean Carb-Up days so you have more flexibility if you're eating out.
- Go on a hike and pack a Ketotarian-friendly picnic.

- Do an evening tea tasting instead of a wine tasting.

- Have a movie marathon and eat Ketotarian-friendly snacks like dark chocolate, olives, and berries.

With a little bit of planning ahead and creativity, the 4-Week Flexible Fasting Plan doesn't have to be a socially isolating experience at all. In fact, it can even connect you with a new community, deepen your friendships, and allow you to bond with your circle over something new and different. And as always, if you're having any criticisms or doubt cast your way, connect with your purpose and stay the course. Who knows, you may inspire the naysayers to change their minds.

Make Food and Fasting Your Friend

Disordered eating and body image issues exist on a spectrum. Many of us struggle with body image issues, yo-yo dieting, and obsessive thoughts about food on a daily basis even if we've never been diagnosed with an eating disorder. This can make us unhappy and straight-up exhausted all. the. time.

If you can relate to that, I want you to remember that this book is all about throwing out the old and welcoming the new. And I'm going to ask you to make a massive perspective shift about food, fasting,

and yourself as well. Because the truth is, you can fast for eighteen hours a night and eat a perfect Ketotarian diet, but in my experience, if your relationship with food and your body is unhealthy, you are not going to enjoy all the goodness the 4-Week Fasting Plan has to offer. In my years of clinical experience, any lifestyle change is more effective when it's born out of self-respect and a healthy relationship with food.

That is why, throughout the course of this book, I want you to make food and fasting your friends and see them for what they are—amazing tools to help you thrive. The key is to eat and fast consciously in loving awareness. Eliminating certain foods that don't make you feel great during this plan is not a way to punish your body, but a way to show yourself deep honor and respect. Love yourself enough to nourish your body with good food medicine. Your body is alive because of brilliant biochemistry, and with each meal, focus on how you can fuel yourself.

Negative and stressful thoughts can be softened by reading or listening to positive things. For example, classical or meditation music, a happy podcast (like that of yours truly), a self-help book, or just silence can be the perfect paths to quieting the mind. Research confirms that we can rewire our brains the more we do something—so make positivity a habit. This tool is not directly measurable, but it is the fertile ground from which all sustainable wellness practices grow.

A GO-TO BREATHING EXERCISE FOR STRESSFUL MOMENTS

When we're stressed and holding in tension, our breath can become shallow—which, unfortunately, only feeds anxiety further. Observing your breath is a fundamental way to bring inner stillness to your day. I recommend conscious breathing to anchor you in the present moment. Whenever you find yourself getting stressed at work or with your family or partner, take a few moments to just breathe naturally and focus on those breaths, letting worries and anxieties diffuse and drift away. If you want a breathing exercise with a little more structure, I recommend the 4-7-8 breath, which is an incredibly simple way to manage stress! Just inhale for 4 seconds, hold your inhale for 7 seconds, and then exhale through the nose for 8 seconds. This breathing exercise was created by Dr. Andrew Weil, the founder of one of the biggest holistic medical centers in the world, and is often described as a "natural tranquilizer for the nervous system."

A word of warning: Effectively managing chronic stress is not just about checking tasks off your "stress management to-do list." In fact, sometimes it requires a massive perspective shift that forces us to stop living in the past or worrying about the future and instead grounds us in the present moment, observing our own thoughts and behavior without judgment. Make self-care a form of self-respect. After many years of working with patients on their stress levels, I can tell you that the true key to befriending your mind and body and decreasing stress really is awareness. We touched on awareness when we talked about mindful eating, but I want you to continue to exercise awareness in all aspects of your life throughout these four weeks. Awareness is like a muscle—you have to use it to make it stronger, and if you don't use it, you lose it.

The thing I love most about awareness is that it's not about fixing a problem or becoming anything, it's just about observing yourself, your thoughts, your reactions to stressors in your life and understanding yourself better. Practice awareness enough and you'll come to see yourself as the observer of your thoughts, not the victim of them.

I often recommend that my patients practice awareness as a way to become more—well, *aware*—of their health choices and negative, repetitive thought patterns—so that they can become more fully present. When you become more aware, you get in touch with who you were created to be, your intrinsic worth, and healthy choices will come much more naturally. When you become aware, you'll be able to drop the shame or rules about food and instead focus on nourishing your body. It is the precipice to the healing of your relationship with your body and with yourself. When you discover that you are deeply worthy of love and care, acts of radiant wellness flow naturally from that space. This is the genesis of sustainable wellness.

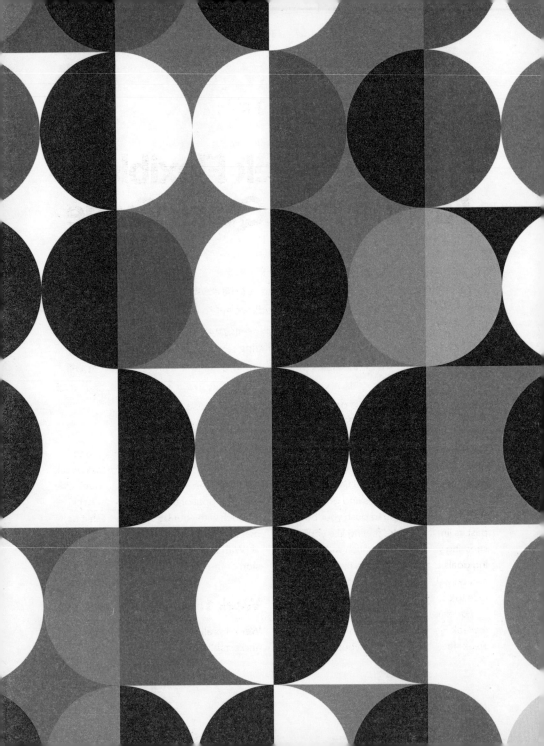

CHAPTER 11

The 4-Week Flexible Fasting Plan Quick Guide

Now that we've talked about all the benefits of the 4-Week Flexible Fasting Plan, why we're doing it, and all the delicious foods we get to nourish ourselves with when we're not fasting, it's time to review exactly what you'll be doing during the four weeks. Use this chapter (and the corresponding recipes and meal plans in Part 4) as your reference sheet and quick guide during the plan. The present chapter will have all the information you need to know about what to eat, when to eat, and which lifestyle practices to focus on during that particular phase of the plan.

Before we dive in, here are a few general points to remember: this is a flexible fasting plan—emphasis on the word *flexible*. While I've outlined general rules and goals for the plan, I never want you to push your body past its limits. If you're feeling like you're stressing your body too much with the fasting goals in this book, listen to your body and do what feels right to you. There's no race to establish metabolic flexibility.

For example, if the first week of the 4-Week Flexible Fasting Plan—the Reset week—feels like a shock to your body and

you're worried about changing it up too soon, repeat the Reset week the next week and then lean into the Recharge week after that. The goal of this plan is to get back in touch with your body, not punish it or make it jump through unnecessary hoops.

With that in mind, here's a distilled version of the 4-Week Flexible Fasting Plan:

Week 1: Reset

Week 1 is all about **resetting your body** and establishing basic **metabolic flexibility**.

We're going to accomplish this through following a **beginner time-restricted feeding plan** and **maintaining a Ketotarian diet**.

Here's what to do this week:

- Fast for **12 hours a day**, which means leaving a gap between dinner and breakfast the next day.

- During your 12-hour eating window, eat as often and as much food as you want. Remember: **Do not restrict calories**.

- During your fasting window, consume only calorie-free, sugar-free liquids like coffee, tea, and water.

- **Eliminate late-night snacking:** Try not to eat for at least 2 hours before bed. This will improve your sleep and make establishing metabolic flexibility easier.

- Follow a **Ketotarian diet plan** as closely as possible. This means you should get:

  - 60 to 75 percent of your calories from fat.

  - 15 to 30 percent of your calories from protein.

  - 5 to 15 percent of your calories from healthy carbohydrates.

- Aim for **20 to 55 grams of net carbs daily**.

- Write down, on paper, your motivations for completing the 4-Week Flexible Fasting Plan. Read that paper anytime you're thinking about breaking a fast early or eating foods that are off the plan.

During Week 1, you may experience symptoms of **sugar withdrawal** and the **keto flu**, which can include fatigue, headache, cravings, nausea, insomnia, irritability, and upset stomach. If you do, try to do the following:

- Drink more water.

- Go for a walk.

- Sleep as much as you need. To prioritize sleep, make sure you're making your bedroom a technology-free zone and avoiding looking at screens at least 1 hour before bed. Then, make sure your bedroom is dark, cool, and quiet. Combined, these factors will all help you sleep more soundly. If you're really having trouble sleeping, try magnesium, l-theanine, melatonin, or chamomile.

Week 1 is meant to ease you into a fasting plan in a way that is gentle and intuitive for your body. I'd recommend avoiding the following during Week 1 and throughout the fasting plan:

- **Over-caffeinating:** It's tempting to hit the espresso shots hard when you're fasting, but I recommend maintaining your normal caffeine intake during the first week of your fast. Too much caffeine can make you hungry, irritable, shaky, and mess with your stress hormones.

- **Cutting calories:** If one of your goals with the 4-Week Flexible Fasting Plan is weight loss, you may be tempted to cut calories right away. Please don't! Your body needs plenty of fuel to adapt to the changes in your eating behavior. Give it what it needs this week and throughout the 4-Week Flexible Fasting Plan and eat until satiety.

- **Over-exercising:** It's awesome to be all in on this plan, and exercise is an important piece of the puzzle. That said, this first week is not the time to sign up for CrossFit or to start training for a triathlon. Instead, go for a walk, do some light exercise, or just maintain your typical level of physical activity.

Your goal during Week 1 is simple: to introduce your body to a gentle fasting plan and a low-carb diet. This will show your body how to burn fat for fuel, something it will need the week to adjust to. This week is all about setting a foundation for metabolic flexibility to prepare your body for the longer fasts in Week 2 and Week 3. That said, you can also expect to observe some immediate benefits, including:

- Weight loss and fat loss

- Reduced sugar cravings and reduced hunger

- Relief from some digestive issues

- Lowered inflammation levels

This week is all about transitioning to fat burning in the gentlest but most efficient way possible. It's important to **follow** **the plan as closely as possible this week**, especially when it comes to your sugar and carbohydrate intake. Even one small hard candy or a few bites of a muffin can sabotage your progress toward becoming an efficient fat-burner, so this is not the week to be laissez-faire about what you eat. Use the meal plans and recipes provided in Part 4 to help you get the right nutrient balance and . . . The good news is that if you're able to stick closely to the plan this week, the next 3 weeks of the plan will be so much easier.

Week 2: Recharge

Week 2 is all about **recharging your metabolism**, which means restoring healthy blood sugar balance and improving heart health and metabolic markers, such as blood lipid levels. To accomplish this, you'll be following an **intermediate time-restricted feeding plan** and introducing an **optional Clean Carb-Up day** once or twice per week.

Here's what to do this week:

- Fast for **14 to 18 hours a day.** I don't give you an exact time frame because this is an *intuitive* fasting plan, so I want you to practice listening to your body.

- During your 6- to 10-hour eating window, eat as much and as often as you want.

- Add in **Clean Carb-Ups days once or twice this week** if you're experiencing any irritability, hunger, or trouble sleeping. That means increasing your net carb intake to 75 to 150 grams of net carbs per day and reducing your healthy fat intake to compensate for this increase.

- On the other days, continue to eat your normal high-fat, low-carbohydrate (fewer than 55 grams net carbs per day) Ketotarian diet.

- **Practice mindful eating.** Take a few deep breaths before you eat and try to limit distractions, such as your phone or the TV.

This week you'll be completing longer fasts, which will require longer periods of time without food. Here are some of my best tips for completing longer fasts and maximizing the benefits of Week 2:

- **Sip on tea:** Organic tea is a great beverage to lean on when you're fasting. It's more interesting to your taste buds than water, has less caffeine than coffee, and contains catechins, compounds that have been linked to a decrease in the hunger hormone ghrelin, meaning it helps make fasting easier.

- **Focus on healthy fats and proteins:** Fats and proteins provide more lasting energy than carbohydrates. This week, make sure you focus on incorporating some kind of healthy fat and clean protein into every meal and even snacks. Try the Smoked Trout and Avocado Rice Bowls (page 234) for dinner or the Almond Chiller (page 192) for an afternoon snack.

- **Try a fasted workout:** Start with low-intensity cardio exercise—I recommend light jogging, walking, or cycling—and slowly increase the intensity of your fasted workouts as your body adjusts.

This week, our moderate fasts will focus on **recharging your metabolism**, which has no doubt suffered from the snack-filled, carb-heavy modern world. This week you'll already have a foundation for metabolic flexibility, which means you can really dive **deeper into ketosis** and make lasting changes in your metabolism. Here are some benefits to keep in mind—and keep you motivated!— throughout Week 2:

- Improved blood sugar balance

- Healthier cardio-metabolic markers, including blood lipids

- Steadier energy levels and a more stable mood

Last week you may have experienced some negative side effects, but this week it's very likely that you'll start to feel better than you have in a long time. If you feel great, skip the Carb-Up days; they're not mandatory and you should use them only if you feel you need them. If you're feeling a little lost at your normal mealtime, try leaning on some Metaphysical Meals and do some journaling exercises or establish a ritual that replaces your normal habit of eating.

Week 3: Renew

This week, you'll be doing your **deepest fasts** of all, which means it's important to focus on reducing stress and making sure you're getting enough food during your eating window. You'll be leaning on mindfulness and other fast-supporting practices this week.

Here's what to do this week:

- Fast for **20 to 22 hours a day, every other day, completing 3 to 4 nonconsecutive Almost-OMAD fasts (see page 82).**

- The other days, fast for 12 hours like you did in Week 1.

- Maintain a **low-carb clean Ketotarian diet** on all days this week for its fasting-mimicking benefits.

- Don't isolate yourself socially: go on a walk, have a movie night, or schedule a Keto-friendly picnic with friends.

- **Consider incorporating MCTs into your routine:** MCTs from foods like coconut oil and ghee can make your fast easier. If you want to get really fancy, add these oils to coffee or tea and drink them before a workout. A great way to add MCTs to your routine is by taking your morning coffee and making it keto (see page 133). Don't forget your electrolytes: this week, drinking just water won't be enough. Deepening your ketosis like we are doing this week can also put you at risk for deficiencies in electrolytes like sodium, magnesium, and potassium. The good news is that this can easily be solved by adding electrolyte supplements or water with a little sea salt to your routine throughout the day.

- **Exercise on your shorter fast days:** Exercise on your lighter fast days. This way, you're not pushing your body to work out after you've been fasting for 20 to 22 hours, and any post-workout hunger will happen during your feeding window.

The longer fasts you'll be doing this week are leaving plenty of time for mechanisms like autophagy and ketosis to really kick into gear. The result is **cellular renewal,** which means long-term benefits like:

- Long-term disease prevention, including autoimmune diseases, neurodegenerative diseases, inflammatory diseases, and lifestyle-related diseases such as cancer, heart disease, and diabetes

- Increased longevity

- Improvements in symptoms of certain chronic diseases

- Increased autophagy, or cellular renewal

- Increased stem cells, needed for body repair

For some, extended fasting can be overwhelming at first. You might be worried about getting lightheaded or not completing your fast. This is normal. If you're feeling stressed, lean on the **stress-management tips,** like decluttering your space and getting into nature. For acute moments of stress, try **4-7-8 breathing** to get your nervous system back on track. You're stronger and more resilient than you think!

Fasting Troubleshooting

If you're having trouble completing your fasts, first ask yourself if you've been eating foods that are helping or hurting your cause. Trust me when I say that if you're following the nutrition plan laid out in this book, fasting will be way easier. The foods I've included here help decrease inflammation, balance blood sugar, and return your leptin levels to a healthy place that lets you easily and intuitively go longer periods of time without food. If you are following the meal plan, try asking yourself the following questions:

- Are you restricting your calories? If so, increase calories during your eating windows.

- Can you add additional veggies, protein, and healthy fats to your plate?

- Are you drinking enough water? Did you forget to add electrolytes?

- Having you been over-exercising? Can you take a day off today or tomorrow?

- Have you been moving your body enough?

- Have you been managing your stress?

- Would a hot cup of herbal tea quell your craving?

- Have you been drinking too much caffeine?

- Have you been sleeping for at least 7 hours a night?

- Have you been turning off your phone, computer, and TV at least an hour before bed?

- If you're feeling amped, stressed, cranky, or anxious, can you do a Clean Carb-Up day tomorrow and see how you feel?

If you've been through this list and you feel that you must break your fast, try some broth, a scoop of no-sugar-added nut butter, or a few spoonfuls of avocado.

Week 4: Rebalance

This week we're focusing on **hormone balance**, which means we'll be going back to a **beginner time-restricted feeding plan** and **incorporating Clean Carb Cycling** to replenish the body's glycogen stores and make sure leptin is in balance.
Here's what to do this week:

- To focus on hormone balance, you'll return to a **12-hour fasting window on all days.**

- You'll also be cycling in and out of our Ketotarian diet plan by experimenting with **2 to 4 Clean Carb-Up days**.

- You should try Clean Carb Cycling if you're experiencing any of the 3 S's:

sleep issues, stalled goals, or sex hormone imbalances.

- On Clean Carb-Up days, add in clean carbs, such as higher-fructose fruits, rice, legumes, and starchy vegetables, so that you are consuming between 75 grams to 150 grams net carbs each day. Two of my favorite Clean Carb-Up day recipes are the Sweet Potato + Nut Butter Stew (page 219) and my Carrot and Lentil Salad (page 196). You should be mindful of adding in Clean Carb-Up days if you have insulin resistance or you are overweight or obese.

If you want to lean more into the **Cyclical Ketotarian plan** this week, here's a quick guide:

- If you're trying to push past a weight loss plateau, do 2 to 4 Carb-Up days.

- If you're trying to balance sex hormones, consider doing 4 Carb-Up days a month—2 on days 1 and 2 of your menstrual cycle and the other 2 on the days following ovulation, such as around days 19 and 20 of your cycle, which is about 5 days after ovulation. Feel free to move these Clean Carb-Up days to any week to sync with your cycle.

- In general, try your heavier workouts on the Carb-Up days, preferably right before your biggest carb meal.

Your goal during Week 4 is to rebalance the most intricate hormones in your system, which means you are tailoring your approach to support:

- Improved thyroid and sex hormone health

- Leptin and ghrelin balance, which means balanced hunger signals

- Healthy melatonin and serotonin production, which means better sleep and a healthier mood

One of the biggest focuses this week is on **cultivating a healthier relationship** with food and with yourself. You can do this by **practicing awareness**—awareness of your thoughts and feelings about food. Ask yourself: What habits were really serving me before this plan and which ones were not? Consider which thought patterns you would like to leave behind and which you want to bring forward.

As you move through this last week of the plan and decide how you're going to incorporate intermittent fasting into your life, listen to that quiet voice inside you, your intuition.

At this point, you'll have established some metabolic flexibility and **you can trust your intuition about what your body needs**. If you feel better eating more carbs, there's absolutely nothing wrong with that. If you enjoy the way you feel on the keto diet long-term, have at it! This week is about slowing down, showing yourself some love, and coming up with a plan that works for you in the long term.

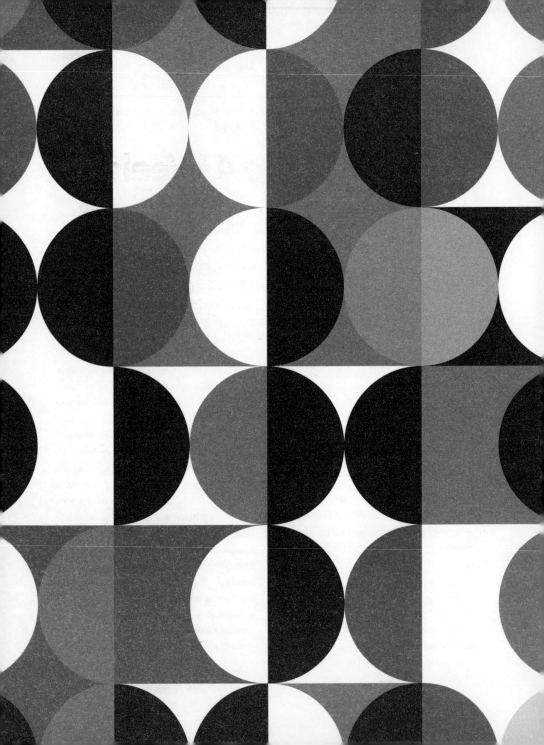

CHAPTER 12

Beyond the 4 Weeks

If you've completed the 4-Week Flexible Fasting Plan, congratulations! You don't need me to tell you what an incredible accomplishment this is. Over these past four weeks, you have established more metabolic flexibility, balanced leptin, decreased inflammation, balanced your blood sugar, worked to restore your gut health, enhanced autophagy, and activated many other healing pathways in your body.

You've learned to stretch and compress your fasting window, Clean Carb Cycle, and have completed fasted and non-fasted workouts. You've taken steps to sleep more soundly and move your body more, and you've worked to decrease chronic stress and cultivate a healthy and supportive community. You've taken longer breaks from eating than maybe ever before in your life. You've stopped eating out of habit and instead connected with your actual physiological hunger signals and hormones. You've taken steps to improve heart health and brain health; increase longevity; maintain a healthy weight; prevent obesity and diabetes; promote a healthy gut and microbiome; and optimize energy levels. You've put your

emotional relationship with food under a microscope, turning it upside down and inside out, and you've figured out what's really there. You've observed how your body feels with different fasting windows and different macronutrient ratios. In just four weeks, you have learned more about your body and your health than many people do in a decade. Heck, more than some people do in their whole lives.

Go ahead and give yourself a huge pat on the back for this. Then feel free to ask me the question on your mind, which I already know is, *Where do we go from here?*

You may not want to hear this, but I'm not going to give you hard-and-fast rules about how to intermittently fast and live your life in the long term. Instead, this is where all your hard work to awaken your intuition about food comes in. In this chapter, I'm going to help you take what you've learned and accomplished during these four weeks and bring it beyond—into your real everyday life. I'm going to teach you how to stay metabolically flexible, for good.

The Metabolic Flexibility Quiz: After the 4-Week Flexible Fasting Plan

Thanks to the 4-Week Flexible Fasting Plan, you've made major strides at correcting underlying health imbalances, established metabolic flexibility, and, most likely, you feel *really good*—probably better than you can remember feeling in a long time.

But how do you know, without a shadow of a doubt, that you've achieved full metabolic flexibility? You take the questionnaire I designed for exactly that purpose, of course. For the following statements, give yourself 1, 2, or 3 points based on how true the statement is for you.

1 = not true at all
2 = somewhat true
3 = definitely true

1. You find yourself snacking a lot and always have an emergency snack on hand.

2. You have difficulty skipping a meal.

3. You have frequent constant cravings for sugar or carbs.

4. You wake up and have breakfast right away.

5. You often find yourself hungry after dinner and eating before bed.

6. The idea of fasting for eighteen hours seems insurmountable.

7. Your energy levels are inconsistent throughout the day; you wake up groggy.

8. The 3 p.m. slump hits you hard.

9. Your brain doesn't work efficiently if you haven't eaten recently; you can't think when you're hungry.

10. You know you lean on caffeine and sugar for energy more than you should.

11. You plan your workouts around your meals.

12. You tend to feel "hangry" or shaky if you don't eat every few hours.

13. You can't work out first thing in the morning without eating first.

14. What you're going to eat and when occupies a lot of your brain space.

15. You often feel hungry right after you eat or within a few hours.

16. When you eat sugar, you don't feel satisfied and instead crave more sugar.

17. You experience anxiety if you have to skip a meal or delay a meal.

18. You rely on carbs for bursts of energy levels.

19. You feel at the mercy of your hunger and food habits; you are not in control.

20. You know that many of your food choices are emotional.

21. You sometimes find yourself eating even when you're not hungry.

22. You sometimes use food as a stress-reliever.

23. Your previous attempts to cut down on sugar have failed.

24. A life without sugar or bread feels scary and depressing.

25. You often experience brain fog or have difficulty concentrating.

Now add up all of your points. Remember, when you first did the quiz, your results revealed whether you were not-so flexible, fairly flexible, or fully flexible. This time, we're going to interpret your results based on how much your score has improved.

Decreased by 10 Points or Fewer

If your score went down by 10 points or fewer, you've still made *major* strides toward metabolic flexibility. If your overall score is still greater than 40, I'd recommend cycling through the entire plan again. Make sure you're experimenting with Carb-Up days, and don't forget about sleep, exercise, and stress management and the key roles they play in metabolic flexibility.

Decreased by 10 to 20 Points

If your score went down by more than 10 points, pat yourself on the back. This is huge progress! Your metabolism has clearly responded well to the plan. If your score is still above 30, I'd still recommend cycling through the plan or repeating the last two weeks. Remember to focus on longer fasts and on adding in MCTs to make sure you're getting deep into ketosis.

Decreased by 20-Plus Points

If your metabolic inflexibility score went down by more than 20 points, it's time to bring out the low-fructose fruit and healthy fats to celebrate. This is an amazing accomplishment, and I have no doubt that you took the Toolbox chapter seriously and didn't neglect your stress levels, exercise, or sleep schedule throughout the plan.

If you don't feel like you've quite reached the promised land when it comes to metabolic flexibility, that's okay. This is about progression, not perfection. Everyone comes into the four weeks from a different place. Some of you will have deeper underlying health imbalances to correct and lifestyle habits to unlearn, while some of you may have already spent considerable time optimizing your well-being, and the 4-Week Flexible Fasting Plan may have just been the cherry on top. Wherever you are, know that your efforts are going a long way toward your overall health and metabolic flexibility.

If you know that you still have some ground to cover before you reach true metabolic flexibility, my suggestion would be to repeat the 4-Week Flexible Fasting Plan. This will allow your body an additional four weeks to reset, recharge, renew, and rebalance. Most likely, you just have some stubborn underlying health imbalances that need a little extra space and time to resolve themselves. The great thing about the 4-Week Flexible Fasting Plan is that—unlike restrictive cleanses, diets, and detoxes—you can repeat it as many times as you need to until you reach your goals.

It doesn't matter how many cycles it takes you to establish metabolic flexibility. The end result is the same—total liberation from cravings, shakiness, and instability in your hunger levels, energy levels, and mood. It's hard to describe just how incredible it feels to establish metabolic flexibility— you have to experience it for yourself.

If you complete the 4-Week Flexible Fasting Plan twice and don't notice measurable improvements in your health and metabolic flexibility, I'd recommend finding an integrative or functional medicine practitioner. I consult with people around the world via webcam at www .drwillcole.com, or you can visit www

.functionalmedicine.org to find a practitioner near you. The 4-Week Flexible Fasting Plan is designed to work for everyone and to correct the most common underlying health issues I see among my patients, but in some cases it takes a highly trained eye to see what's holding you back from feeling your best. In my functional medicine practice, I use diagnostic testing and analysis that's rarely done in conventional settings to uncover the hidden causes of metabolic inflexibility. I take great pride in delivering personalized health guidance to patients as well as in providing an environment that supports and inspires them. Unlike conventional doctor visits that last an average of seventeen minutes, I often spend over an hour at a time with my patients, listening, asking questions, and acting like a private investigator to uncover the root cause of their health issues.

If you do feel like you've established metabolic flexibility, congratulations! I'm so glad the plan worked so well for you. You may feel more energized and stronger than you have in years. You may feel an amazing sense of liberation—both mental and physical. You may feel more satisfied after each meal and like you're no longer a victim of your metabolism, cravings, and imbalanced microbiome and inflammation levels. If you're experiencing these benefits, I want you to lean in and enjoy every second of your hard-earned good health. It's because of your willingness to try something new and get out of your comfort zone that you get to experience these benefits.

So now that begs the question: What comes next?

How to Stay Metabolically Flexible for Life

Moving forward, I do recommend that you keep up with some type of intermittent fasting plan. Metabolic flexibility is, after all, like a muscle—if you don't use it, you'll lose it. The good news is, now that you're metabolically flexible, fasting and cyclical low-carb eating will come naturally to you. Now that you can burn fat and sugar for fuel and you've lowered inflammation, balanced blood sugar, and improved your gut health, you won't be all that tempted to return to many of your old habits. You'll want to continue to chase the feeling of steadiness and freedom you've achieved.

As you moved through the plan, you probably noticed that on some days and weeks you felt better than on others. If there was a part of the plan that appealed to you, worked with your schedule, and made you feel good, make that your long-term plan. Did shorter fasts and a Ketotarian diet feel amazing to your body? Keep that up. Did you feel better with longer fasts but felt too fatigued without Clean Carb-Up days? Keep that up. As long as you feel good, keep it up. Basically, keep up with whatever felt good, and trust

your body to tell you if something needs adjusting down the line.

Whether you're making your own meal or eating out, follow these basic "ketotarianisms":

1. Eat real food.

2. Keep your carbs low.

3. Keep your healthy fats high.

4. If you eat a non-starchy vegetable, add some healthy fats.

5. If you eat a healthy fat, add some non-starchy vegetables.

6. Eat when you are hungry.

7. Eat until you are satiated.

Don't forget the Clean Carb Cycle for sleep optimization, sex hormone balance, or stalled goals. Use the Ketotarian food list as your foundation, but when it comes to food and drinks that you avoided during the plan, you may find that you don't actually miss them in the way you thought you would. If you want to bring back a few of your favorite foods, pick the ones you missed the most, then add them in, one by one, and observe how you feel. Try to keep a week in between add-ins so you have enough time to see how those foods affect your health.

So, for example, you may miss red wine, goat cheese, and sourdough bread the most. Add them back in, in moderation and one-by-one over three weeks, and see if you can feel as good as you did during the plan while still eating those foods. If the answer is no, consider eliminating them permanently. If the answer is yes, eat them in moderation and observe how you feel. As you quiet the noise of imbalance in your body and gain metabolic flexibility, the still, small voice of your intuition will be clear and resolute.

You may be thinking, "Slow down, Dr. Cole! That's a lot of responsibility to put in my hands!" It is, but now that you've established metabolic flexibility, you can trust your own body to send you the right signals. At the end of the day, you know your body better than I ever could.

If you're still unclear about which fasting plan is right for you in the long term, I recommend aiming to fast for at least 12 hours every night as you did on Weeks 1 and 4; also aim to maintain a flexible Ketotarian diet as much as you can, adding in Carb-Up days when you see fit. Then, anywhere from a few times a week to a few times a month, extend your fast for 18 to 22 hours.

As you transition back into normal life, keep the metabolic flexibility quiz on hand. If your needs ever change and you're starting to become metabolically inflexible again, fall back on the 4-Week Flexible Fasting Plan and simply cycle through the four weeks. I love to do it seasonally to reset, recharge, renew, and rebalance my body, but you can do it any four weeks out of the year. If there was a

week of the plan that you found particularly effective, follow that protocol for two weeks or the full four weeks. It's called the *flexible* fasting plan for a reason.

That's one of the things I love most about intermittent fasting. It's not about dogma or labels or fitting into just one nutrition or food philosophy. Instead, it's all about finding a way of eating that works for you, your schedule, and your lifestyle.

Basking in the Light of Food Peace

Over the last four weeks you've turned everything you know about eating (and not eating!) upside down. You've broken habits that have been with you for years or even decades and, for some of you, for as long as you can remember. In this last section of the book, I want to make sure we don't brush over just how brave you were for doing this. Habits, especially those surrounding food, can make us feel safe and help us cope, and we often use them to regulate our emotions. Untangling ourselves from these habits can be downright scary. But, nevertheless, you persevered.

By leaving the antiquated food rules and restrictions in the past, you've been able to quiet the noise and get in touch with your intuition. You've brought your lifestyle down to the foundation and rebuilt it in love for yourself. Ask yourself: What do I really need to feel good? What is my body really trying to tell me? How can I give it space and reconnect it with an eating style that is more in line with how my body was beautifully designed to function—not just on a metabolic level, but on a cellular one as well?

Thanks to your bravery, strength, and diligent work, by the end of the fasting plan, the once muffled voice inside you is clear and certain. Now that you are metabolically flexible, you can exhale, sit in stillness, and know what you need to thrive.

In the last four weeks, you have been liberating your brain from worrying and stressing about food and being a victim of your metabolic inflexibility and underlying health imbalances. And now that you've reconnected with your body, fasting won't feel so burdensome. In fact, it'll come naturally and easily, with a grace and lightness so radiant you could cry with joy to be free from dieting dogma. Unbound from the shackles of food shame, you may sit down for your first meal a few months from now and realize, wow, you just fasted for eighteen hours and didn't even realize it. You may get to a place where you wake up in the morning and your body tells you, "This morning, I'm hungry," so you eat a wonderful nourishing breakfast. Then, the next day that voice tells you, "No, I'm not hungry yet," and so you continue with your fast.

Eating only when you're truly hungry seems painfully simple, but getting to a place where your body tells you what to eat—instead of what your cravings, emo-

tions, or society's arbitrary food rules are telling you—is the real goal of this book, and it's not an easy goal to accomplish.

Eating only when you are truly hungry? Eating only until you're full? Never feeling like you're restricting or punishing yourself? That, my friend, is food peace.

In the end, this book isn't really about fasting for eighteen hours a day or eating a perfect low-carb diet, it's about balancing your body so that you can listen to it, knowing that it won't lead you astray. That means if you don't feel like fasting one day, you simply . . . don't. Once you've established metabolic flexibility, you can trust your body to skip that day and pick it up the next.

A lot of people live in fear that they will fall off the wagon, that one broken fast will spiral and lead to a lifetime of poor food and lifestyle choices. And when you're metabolically inflexible, this is not necessarily untrue. Trying to eat healthy while being metabolically inflexible is like trying to keep a dam from breaking every single day, trying to keep it together while cracks form and water escapes over the top and the sides. Making healthy choices when you're metabolically inflexible feels utterly arduous and punitive, and you have to be "perfect" or everything will fall apart. Unfortunately, the result of this is a lifetime of cravings, shame, and denying yourself, feeling perpetually dissatisfied and afraid of what will happen if you slip up.

But when you've established metabolic flexibility, making healthy lifestyle choices will feel like you're flowing downstream safely in your boat of peace that you've built yourself. When you've found food peace, you can trust your body to do right by you, and you know that its natural instinct is always to return to a healthy way of eating and living.

I would describe the feeling of food peace as a vibrant stillness and knowingness, the absence of obsessive shaming thoughts and anxiety about what you're going to eat and when. You feel like you're the creator of your own lifestyle instead of the victim of it. This allows you to really focus on things like your work, your family, and being present and enjoying your life. Instead of having thoughts about what to eat and when occupying your head at all hours of the day and night, things feel . . . simple. Straightforward.

Food peace is truly sustainable wellness that flows from realizing your intrinsic worth and is born out of self-respect. When you realize that you are a beautiful creation that is loved and are able to love yourself in return, you naturally do acts of radiant wellness. When you learn to love feeling great more than you want to eat the food that will diminish how you feel, that's food peace. And if you eat something that doesn't serve you, you don't shame yourself. You eat it, are conscious of how it makes you feel, learn from it, and move on. Wellness imbued with grace and lightness. This is food peace. This is intuitive eating and the heart of *Intuitive Fasting*.

And now for the most important question I will ask in this book: Now that you have all this extra clarity and freedom, what are you going to do with it?

This book is about establishing metabolic flexibility, connecting with your intuition, and finding peace with food, yes. But it's also about taking advantage of those dissipating worries about food and channeling your newfound capacity and energy elsewhere.

Now that you've achieved food peace, what will you spend that time creating, doing, or thinking about instead? The truth is, worrying about food all the time is exhausting and, honestly, boring. You are meant for greater things.

So many people are kept back from who they were created to be, bound by their imbalance, divorced from their intuition. Like a flower that has never bloomed, stuck in proverbial winter.

May you, who has remained dormant until, now bloom wildly.

Will you work to be more creative, more present, more thoughtful? Will you listen better, concentrate deeper, and be more empathetic? Will you channel that energy into your career, your partner, your children? You can't pour from an empty cup.

We've spent the last four weeks resetting, recharging, renewing, and rebalancing your cup. Now take that newfound energy, steadiness, and peace of mind out in the world and see what you can do.

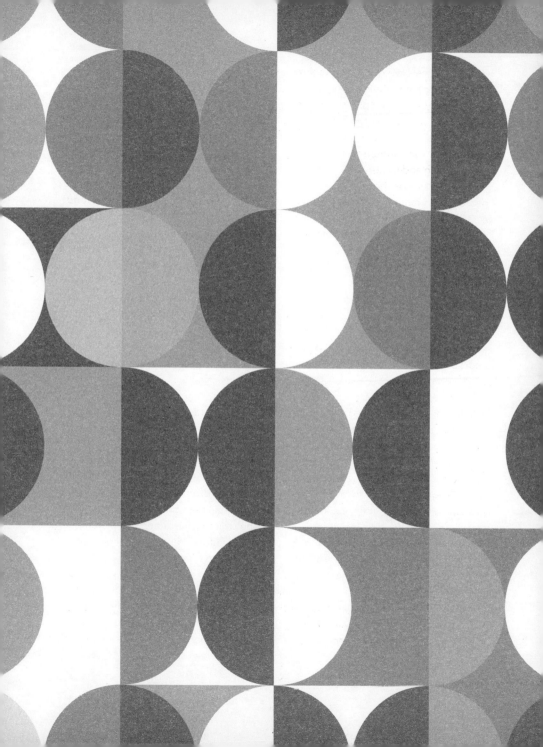

PART FOUR

Intuitive Fasting Recipes and Meal Plan

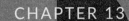

CHAPTER 13

Intuitive Fasting
Manifested: The Recipes

Note: First, Second, and Third Meals can be used interchangeably, keeping in mind that for longer fasts in Week 3, it's best to use a gentle Break-a-Fast option as your first meal.

Ketotarian 4-Week Meal Plan

WEEK 1 Body Reset: 12:12 Fast (Ketotarian)

NUTRIENT GUIDELINES PER DAY: FATS: 60–75%; PROTEINS: 15–30%; CARBS: 5–15%; NET CARBS: <55G

	Sunday	Monday	Tuesday	Wednesday	Thursday	Friday	Saturday
	1391 Calories; 75% Fat, 18% Protein, 7% Carbs; 26g Net Carbs	1512 Calories; 75% Fat, 16% Protein, 9% Carbs; 35g Net Carbs	1694 Calories; 77% Fat, 13% Protein, 10% Carbs; 43g Net Carbs	1624 Calories; 73% Fat, 15% Protein, 12% Carbs; 48g Net Carbs	1406 Calories; 68% Fat, 24% Protein, 8% Carbs; 29g Net Carbs	1569 Calories; 72% Fat, 17% Protein, 11% Carbs; 41g Net Carbs	1557 Calories; 68% Fat, 22% Protein, 10% Carbs; 38g Net Carbs
First Meal	Almond Chiller (p. 192)	Mini Broccoli and "Cheese" Frittata (p. 192). Serve with ⅓ cup strawberries.	Overnight Lemon-Raspberry Chia Pudding (p. 193)	Skillet Eggs with Spinach (p. 189)	Fresh Ginger Pumpkin Bisque (p. 186). Serve with 2 hard-boiled eggs.	Cream Cheese with Salmon Wrap-Ups (p. 194)	Escarole-Parsnip Soup (p. 185)
Second Meal	Grilled Halibut on Tzatziki Greens (p. 209). Serve with ¼ cup toasted walnuts.	Kale, Brussels Sprout, and Blueberry Salad (p. 255)	Chilled Sweet Pea + Avocado Soup (p. 210)	Smashed Bean Wraps (p. 211)	Chicken, Cabbage, and Sunflower Seed Salad (p. 212)	Arugula-Grapefruit Salad (p. 213)	Walnut and Chicken–Stuffed Celery (p. 214)
Snack	Eggs with Hot Pepper Oil (p. 264)	Creamy Herb Veggie Dip (p. 264)	8 flaxseed crackers with 2 tablespoons almond butter	Blueberry-Matcha Smoothie (p. 265)	Salted Dark Chocolate–Almond Bark (p. 267)	⅓ cup roasted almonds	Green Cucumber Smoothie (p. 190)
Third Meal	Taco Cauliflower Bowl (p. 235)	Turmeric-Rubbed Chicken (p. 236). Serve with Cashew-Ginger Bok Choy (p. 262).	Spinach + Ricotta Portobello Caps (p. 237). Serve with Pepperoncini Tomato Salad (p. 256).	Lemon Chicken (p. 238). Serve with Roasted Carrots with Jalapeño-Pecan Salsa (p. 263).	Skewered Tuna with Avocado Salad Salsa (p. 212)	Poached Eggs with Tarragon Sauce and Asparagus (p. 240)	Homestyle Meatloaf and Roasted Beans (p. 241)

WEEK 2 Metabolism Recharge: Daily 14–18 Hour Fasts (Includes 2 Carb-Up Days)

NUTRIENT GUIDELINES PER DAY: FATS: 60–75%; (CARB-UP: 65%); PROTEINS: 15–30%; (CARB-UP: 15%); CARBS: 5–15%; (CARB-UP: 20%); NET CARBS: 5 DAYS: <55G (KETO DAYS) AND 2 DAYS: 75–150G (CARB-UP DAYS)

	Sunday	Monday	Tuesday	Wednesday	Thursday	Friday	Saturday
	1607 Calories; 79% Fat, 16% Protein, 6% Carbs; 23g Net Carbs	Carb-Up Day 1554 Calories; 70% Fat, 11% Protein, 19% Carbs; 76g Net Carbs	1536 Calories; 72% Fat, 19% Protein, 9% Carbs; 33g Net Carbs	1308 Calories; 71% Fat, 17% Protein, 12% Carbs; 37g Net Carbs	Carb-Up Day 1584 Calories; 69% Fat, 12% Protein, 19% Carbs; 75g Net Carbs	1297 Calories; 70% Fat, 20% Protein, 10% Carbs; 32g Net Carbs	1413 Calories; 79% Fat, 14% Protein, 7% Carbs; 24g Net Carbs
First Meal	Kale Caesar Salad with Eggs (p. 195)	Carrot and Lentil Salad (p. 196). Serve with Pineapple Smoothie (p. 266).	Lemon-Caper Tuna Salad with Cucumber "Chips" (p. 197)	Greens in Ginger Broth (p. 191). Serve with 2 large soft-boiled eggs.	Fresh Dill, Shrimp, and Penne Salad (p. 198) sprinkled with 2 tablespoons toasted pine nuts.	Middle Eastern Spiced Beef on Carrot Spirals (p. 199)	Lox Deviled Eggs with Spinach (p. 200)
Snack	Coconut Lime Smoothie (p. 265) Or ¼ cup toasted macadamia nuts	Spicy Almond Butter Dip (p. 268). Serve with 2 large carrots cut into sticks.	Yogurt Bowls with Cinnamon Chia Berries (p. 269) Or Cocoa-Covered Almond Fat Bombs (p. 271)	⅓ cup toasted walnuts Or ¼ cup fresh blueberries	Strawberry-Spirulina Smoothie (p. 266). Serve with Pickled Carrot Sticks (p. 258).	Avocado "Toasts" (p. 270) Or ⅓ cup fresh blackberries	Almond Chiller (p. 192) Or ¼ cup toasted almonds
Second Meal	Chicken and Mushrooms with Balsamic-Wine Reduction (p. 215). Serve with sautéed zucchini noodles.	Tarragon Beet Salad with Cream Cheese "Croutons" (p. 216). Serve with ½ avocado, sliced.	Spicy Veggie Scramble (p. 217)	Buttery Sea Scallops on Garlic Snow Peas (p. 218). Serve with Jicama and Fresh Mint Salad (p. 257).	Sweet Potato + Nut Butter Stew (p. 219)	Tempeh-Walnut Bowls (p. 220)	Caprese Zoodle Salad (p. 221)

WEEK 3 Cellular Renewal: Every Other Day 20–22 Hour Fast Almost-OMAD (12:12 Ketotarian Fast on the Other Days)

NUTRIENT GUIDELINES PER DAY: FATS: 60–75%; PROTEINS: 15–30%; CARBS: 5–15%; NET CARBS: <55G

	Sunday	Monday	Tuesday	Wednesday	Thursday	Friday	Saturday
	Almost-OMAD Day 1204 Calories; 78% Fat, 14% Protein, 8% Carbs; 24g Net Carbs	1635 Calories; 68% Fat, 21% Protein, 11% Carbs; 43g Net Carbs	Almost-OMAD Day 1213 Calories; 73% Fat, 17% Protein, 10% Carbs; 30g Net Carbs	1599 Calories; 71% Fat, 18% Protein, 11% Carbs; 42g Net Carbs	Almost-OMAD Day 1242 Calories; 73% Fat, 16% Protein, 11% Carbs; 33g Net Carbs	1519 Calories; 73% Fat, 18% Protein, 9% Carbs; 35g Net Carbs	Almost-OMAD Day 1281 Calories; 78% Fat, 14% Protein, 8% Carbs; 26g Net Carbs
First Meal/ Break-a-Fast	Green Cucumber Smoothie (p. 190)	Beef Roll Ups (p. 201)	Tomato-Arugula Soup (p. 183)	Keto Cinnamon Granola Cereal (p. 202)	Creamy Roasted Pepper Soup (p. 184)	Tropical Yogurt Bowl (p. 202)	2 hard-boiled eggs with 1½ cups almond milk
Second Meal	Two poached eggs served over Broccoli-Mushroom Roast with Sesame Seeds (p. 260). Serve with ½ small avocado and ¼ cup toasted cashews.	Egg, Nut, and Cheese Bento Box (p. 222)	Grilled Chicken Thigh (p. 222). Serve with Grilled Eggplant with Tomato Relish (p. 261) topped with 2 tablespoons toasted pine nuts.	Coconut Thai Shrimp (p. 223)	Dijon Chicken with Green Onion Cauliflower (p. 224). Serve with 1 large clementine.	Deviled Egg Long-Leaf Wraps (p. 225)	Rustic Fish Stew (p. 188). Serve with spinach salad snack
Snack	Crackers with Chive Cheese Spread (p. 271). Serve with ¼ cup fresh raspberries.	Strawberry-Spirulina Smoothie (p. 266)	Fruit Yogurt Cup (p. 270)	Blueberry-Matcha Smoothie (p. 265)	2 Cocoa-Covered Almond Fat Bombs (p. 271)	8 flaxseed crackers with 2 tablespoons almond butter	Marinated Cheese and Olives with Melon and Cucumber (p. 272)
Third Meal	Fast	Grilled Salmon with Fresh Orange + Chia Seed Salsa (p. 242)	Fast	Veggie Frittata with Lemon-Splashed Spring Greens (p. 243)	Fast	Spicy Sauced Beef Tips (p. 244). Serve with mashed turnips.	Fast

WEEK 4 Hormone Rebalance: Daily 12:12 Hour Fasts (Includes Days 1–4 Ketotarian & Days 5–7 Carb-Up Days)

NUTRIENT GUIDELINES PER DAY: FATS: 60–75%; (CARB-UP: 65%); PROTEINS: 15–30%; (CARB-UP: 15%); CARBS: 5–15%; (CARB-UP: 20%); NET CARBS: 4 DAYS: <55G (KETO DAYS) AND 3 DAYS: 75–150G (CARB-UP DAYS)

	Sunday	Monday	Tuesday	Wednesday	Thursday	Friday	Saturday
	1575 Calories; 73% Fat, 20% Protein, 7% Carbs; 27g Net Carbs	1487 Calories; 74% Fat, 16% Protein, 10% Carbs; 36g Net Carbs	1739 Calories; 74% Fat, 15% Protein, 11% Carbs; 50g Net Carbs	1459 Calories; 76% Fat, 17% Protein, 7% Carbs; 26g Net Carbs	Carb-Up Day 1665 Calories; 66% Fat, 14% Protein, 20% Carbs; 82g Net Carbs	Carb-Up Day 1613 Calories; 66% Fat, 14% Protein, 20% Carbs; 79g Net Carbs	Carb-Up Day 1827 Calories; 67% Fat, 14% Protein, 19% Carbs; 86g Net Carbs
First Meal	Crispy Trout with Buttery Shallots and Arugula (p. 203). Serve with 1 cup mixed berries.	Mushroom-Spinach Mini Quiche (p. 204)	Blackberry-Spinach Smoothie (p. 182). Serve with ¼ cup of your favorite nuts.	Zucchini-Asparagus Hash (p. 205)	Avocado + Grapefruit with Coconut Topping (p. 206)	Natto-Rice Bowls (p. 207)	Sweet Potato Patties with Spicy Yogurt (p. 252)
Second Meal	Cauliflower "Tabbouleh" (p. 226)	Beef Patties, Sugar Snaps, and Horse-radish Aioli (p. 227)	Creamy Mustard and Egg Chop Salad (p. 228)	Curried Tuna Salad Wraps (p. 229)	Minted Chickpea Salad (p. 230)	Lentil Rotini and Aspar-agus Salad (p. 231)	Kidney Bean and Egg Salad (p. 232)
Snack	Avocado "Toasts" (p. 270)	Coconut Lime Smoothie (p. 265)	Creamy Herb Veggie Dip (p. 264).	Salted Dark Chocolate–Almond Bark (p. 267)	Spicy Almond Butter Dip (p. 268). Serve with ½ cup cucumber slices.	Lox-Stuffed Cucumber (p. 273). Serve with 1 large clem-entine.	Pineapple Smoothie (p. 266)
Third Meal	Herbed-Ghee Marinated Chicken with Broccoli (p. 245)	Stuffed Squash with Cream Cheese (p. 246). Serve with Greens and Berry Salad with Chia Seed Dress-ing (p. 259).	Sheet Pan Pecan-Crusted Cod and Carrots (p. 247). Serve with Arugula Salad (p. 258).	Walnut Por-tobellos in Sage Butter (p. 248)	Spinach-Artichoke Turmeric Rice (p. 249)	Sesame Thai Toss with Citrus-Nut Butter Sauce (p. 250)	Catfish with Rustic Creole Sauce (p. 251)

CODE

(V) Vegan

(VT) Vegetarian

(VQ) Vegaquarian

(VV) Vegavore

(CU) Carb-Up

BREAK-A-FAST

FIRST MEAL

SECOND MEAL

THIRD MEAL

SNACKS AND SIDES

BONUS

Blackberry-Spinach Smoothie

SERVES 1 • TOTAL TIME: 5 MINUTES

- 1 cup baby spinach
- ½ cup frozen blackberries
- ½ avocado, pitted and peeled
- 1 cup unsweetened almond milk
- 2 tablespoons hemp protein powder
- 1 tablespoon flaxseed oil
- Liquid stevia (optional)

In a blender, combine spinach, blackberries, avocado, almond milk, protein powder, and flaxseed oil. Cover and blend until smooth. If desired, blend in a few drops of liquid stevia.

Nutrition Information (per serving):

Calories 401
Carbohydrate 31g
(Fiber 16g, Sugars 11g)
Fat 32g (Saturated Fat 3.5g)
Protein 12g

Cholesterol 0mg
Sodium 236mg
Macros: 73% Fat, 12% Protein, 15% Carbs
Net Carbs: 15g

Tomato-Arugula Soup

SERVES 2 • PREP: 5 MINUTES • COOK: 20 MINUTES

3 tablespoons olive oil, divided

½ cup finely chopped green bell pepper

⅓ cup thinly sliced carrots

1 (14.5-ounce) can diced tomatoes

2 cups chicken bone broth*

1 cup arugula leaves

Kosher salt and black pepper

1 tablespoon chopped fresh chives

1. Heat 1 tablespoon of oil in a medium saucepan over medium heat. Add the bell peppers and carrots and cook for 4 to 5 minutes or until tender crisp. Add the tomatoes and broth. Bring to a boil over high heat, reduce the heat, cover, and simmer for 15 minutes.

2. Remove from heat and stir in the arugula and remaining 2 tablespoons of oil. Add salt and pepper to taste.

3. Divide between 2 bowls and sprinkle evenly with the chives.

* Note: To make this vegetarian, use vegetable broth.

Nutrition Information (per serving):

Calories 283

Carbohydrate 16g

(Fiber 5g, Sugars 7g)

Fat 22g (Saturated Fat 2.5g)

Protein 12g

Cholesterol 5mg

Sodium 589mg

Macros: 69% Fat, 16% Protein, 15% Carbs

Net Carbs: 11g

Creamy Roasted Pepper Soup

SERVES 2 • PREP: 10 MINUTES • COOK: 25 MINUTES

2 large red or green bell peppers

1½ cups chicken bone broth*

½ teaspoon dried thyme

⅓ cup chopped fresh cilantro or parsley, divided

1 cup full-fat coconut milk

salt and black pepper

1. Line a baking sheet with foil. Preheat the broiler.

2. Cut the peppers in half lengthwise and remove stems, seeds, and membranes. Flatten with the palm of your hand. Place cut-side down on the prepared baking sheet. Broil 2 to 3 inches from the heat source for 7 minutes or until completely blistered, turning occasionally.

3. Remove from the oven and let stand 5 minutes or until cool enough to handle and slip peels off.

4. Place the peppers in a medium saucepan with the broth and thyme. Bring to a boil, reduce heat, and simmer, uncovered, for 15 minutes. Stir in the cilantro, reserving 1 tablespoon. Remove the pot from the heat.

5. Working in two batches, place in a blender, secure with the lid, cover with a clean towel, and puree until smooth. Return the blended soup to the saucepan and add the coconut milk. Over medium heat, cook for 2 to 3 minutes to heat through. Season with salt and pepper to taste.

6. Divide between 2 bowls and sprinkle evenly with the remaining tablespoon of cilantro.

Nutrition Information (per serving):

Calories 295

Carbohydrate 12g

(Fiber 4g, Sugars 4g)

Fat 24g (Saturated Fat 21.4g)

Protein 11g

Cholesterol 0mg

Sodium 253mg

Macros: 75% Fat, 15% Protein, 10% Carbs

Net Carbs: 8g

* Note: To make this vegan keto, use vegetable broth.

Escarole-Parsnip Soup

SERVES 2 • PREP: 5 MINUTES • COOK: 20 MINUTES

2 tablespoons olive oil, divided

¾ cup chopped parsnips

2 cups chicken bone broth or vegetable broth*

8 ounces escarole, chopped

salt

2 ounces vegan feta cheese, crumbled

2 hard-boiled eggs, peeled and chopped

1. In a medium saucepan, heat 1 tablespoon of oil over medium heat. Add the parsnips and cook for 5 minutes or until the parsnips begin to soften, stirring occasionally. Add the broth and bring to a boil over high heat. Reduce the heat, cover, and simmer for 10 minutes or until parsnips are tender.

2. Add the escarole, return to a simmer, and cook until the escarole is almost tender, about 5 minutes.

3. Remove from the heat. Season with salt to taste.

4. Divide between 2 bowls, top with equal amounts of the feta and egg, and drizzle evenly with the remaining tablespoon of oil.

* Note: To make this vegetarian, use vegetable broth.

Nutrition Information (per serving):

Calories 362

Carbohydrate 17g

(Fiber 6g, Sugars 2.9g)

Fat 27g (Saturated Fat 10.6g)

Protein 18g

Cholesterol 186mg

Sodium 601mg

Macros: 68% Fat, 20% Protein, 12% Carbs

Net Carbs: 11g

Fresh Ginger Pumpkin Bisque

SERVES 4 • PREP: 6 MINUTES • COOK: 25 MINUTES

2 tablespoons ghee or olive oil

1 cup sliced carrots

2 cups chicken bone broth or vegetable broth*

1 (15-ounce) can pumpkin puree

1 teaspoon curry powder

½ teaspoon ground cumin

1 cup full-fat coconut milk

2 teaspoons grated fresh ginger

2 to 4 drops liquid stevia, or to taste

¼ cup chopped fresh chives

½ cup unsweetened plain vegan yogurt

1. Heat a large saucepan over medium-high heat until hot. Add the ghee. When melted, add the carrots and cook for 5 minutes or until beginning to lightly brown, stirring frequently. Add the broth, pumpkin, curry powder, cumin, and coconut milk. Bring to a boil, reduce heat, cover, and simmer for 20 minutes or until the carrots are tender, stirring occasionally.

2. Remove from the heat. Stir in the ginger and stevia. Use an immersion blender directly in the pot to blend the soup (or working in batches, place in a blender, secure with lid, cover with a towel, and puree until smooth).

3. Serve topped with chives and yogurt.

* Note: To make this vegan keto, use vegetable broth.

Nutrition Information (per serving):

Calories 266

Carbohydrate 15g

(Fiber 7g, Sugars 5g)

Fat 22g (Saturated Fat 15.1g)

Protein 9g

Cholesterol 14mg

Sodium 190mg

Macros: 73% Fat, 14% Protein, 13% Carbs

Net Carbs: 8g

Mediterranean Eggplant Stew

SERVES 2 • PREP: 10 MINUTES • COOK: 25 MINUTES

3 tablespoons avocado oil, divided

¾ cup coarsely chopped green bell pepper

8 ounces eggplant, cut into ¾-inch cubes

1 crookneck squash or zucchini (about 6 ounces), coarsely chopped

1½ cups grape tomatoes, halved

12 pitted kalamata olives

½ teaspoon dried fennel seeds

¼ cup chopped fresh basil, divided

Kosher salt

4 ounces vegan mozzarella cheese, shredded

1. Heat 1 tablespoon of the oil in a large saucepan over medium-high heat. Add the bell peppers and cook for 4 minutes or until peppers are tender crisp. Stir in the eggplant, squash, tomatoes, olives, and fennel seeds. Bring to a boil, reduce heat, cover, and simmer for 20 to 25 minutes or until bell peppers are tender.

2. Remove from the heat, stir in 3 tablespoons of the basil and the remaining 2 tablespoons of oil. Add salt to taste. Let stand, covered, 10 minutes to absorb flavors.

3. Divide between 2 shallow bowls, sprinkle cheese evenly over all, and top with the remaining tablespoon of basil.

Nutrition Information (per serving):

Calories 473

Carbohydrate 25g

(Fiber 7g, Sugars 9.8g)

Fat 42g (Saturated Fat 13.8g)

Protein 6g

Cholesterol 0mg

Sodium 623mg

Macros: 80% Fat, 5% Protein, 15% Carbs

Net Carbs: 18g

Rustic Fish Stew

SERVES 2 • PREP: 5 MINUTES • COOK: 16 MINUTES

2 tablespoons olive oil

1 cup coarsely chopped green bell pepper

1 cup chopped turnip root

1 (14.5-ounce) can diced tomatoes

½ teaspoon dried thyme

2 tablespoons ghee

¼ cup chopped fresh parsley, divided

½ teaspoon kosher salt

8-ounce cod fillet, rinsed and cut into 1-inch cubes

1. In a large saucepan, heat the oil over medium heat. When hot, add the bell pepper and cook 5 minutes or until beginning to lightly brown, stirring frequently.

2. Add the turnip, tomatoes, 1 cup water, and the thyme. Bring to a boil over high heat, reduce heat, cover, and simmer for 8 to 10 minutes or until the turnip is tender.

3. Add the ghee, all but 1 tablespoon of the parsley, and the salt and stir until well blended. Add the fish and stir *very gently*. Bring to a boil over high heat, reduce heat, cover, and simmer for 3 minutes or until the fish is opaque in the center. Do not stir. Remove from the heat. Cover and let stand for 10 minutes to absorb flavors.

4. Divide between 2 bowls and sprinkle with the remaining 1 tablespoon of parsley.

Nutrition Information (per serving):

Calories 398

Carbohydrate 17g

(Fiber 5g, Sugars 10g)

Fat 29g (Saturated Fat 10.4g)

Protein 23g

Cholesterol 71mg

Sodium 582mg

Macros: 65% Fat, 23% Protein, 12% Carbs

Net Carbs: 12g

Skillet Eggs with Spinach

SERVES 2 • PREP: 5 MINUTES • COOK: 5 MINUTES

2 tablespoons ghee

2 teaspoons fresh lemon juice

¼ teaspoon chili powder

9 ounces (about 5½ cups) fresh spinach

Kosher salt and black pepper

4 large eggs

½ cup chopped tomatoes

1. In a large skillet, heat the ghee over medium-high heat. When ghee has melted, remove 1 tablespoon and place in a small bowl with the lemon juice and chili powder. Set aside.

2. To the remaining ghee in the skillet, add the spinach and ¼ teaspoon salt; cook 1 minute until just beginning to wilt, using two utensils to toss as you would a stir-fry.

3. Make 4 wells in the spinach. Carefully break 1 egg into each well. Cook for 3 to 4 minutes or until the egg whites are set.

4. Remove from heat. Drizzle with the reserved ghee mixture, sprinkle with tomatoes, and season lightly with salt and pepper to taste.

Nutrition Information (per serving):

Calories 300
Carbohydrate 8g
(Fiber 4g, Sugars 2g)
Fat 24g (Saturated Fat 11.6g)
Protein 17g

Cholesterol 394mg
Sodium 490mg
Macros: 72% Fat, 22% Protein, 6% Carbs
Net Carbs: 4g

Green Cucumber Smoothie

SERVES 1 • PREP: 5 MINUTES

¾ cup unsweetened almond milk

½ cup baby spinach

½ cup coarsely chopped seedless cucumber

¼ cup frozen cubed honeydew melon

2 tablespoon fresh mint leaves

1 tablespoon fresh lemon juice

1 tablespoon hemp protein powder

1½ teaspoons spirulina powder

4 teaspoons coconut oil

Sea salt

Liquid stevia (optional)

In a blender, combine the almond milk, baby spinach, cucumber, melon, mint, lemon juice, protein powder, spirulina powder, coconut oil, and a pinch of sea salt. Cover and blend until smooth. If desired, blend in a few drops of liquid stevia.

Nutrition Information (per serving):

Calories 266

Carbohydrate 13g

(Fiber 4g, Sugars 5g)

Fat 22g (Saturated Fat 16g)

Protein 9g

Cholesterol 0mg

Sodium 519mg

Macros: 73% Fat, 13% Protein, 14% Carbs

Net Carbs: 9g

Greens in Ginger Broth

SERVES 2 • PREP: 5 MINUTES • COOK: 11 MINUTES

2 tablespoons toasted sesame oil

1 tablespoon grated fresh ginger

2 cups vegetable broth

1 tablespoon coconut aminos

1 teaspoon fresh lime juice

4 cups baby spinach

2 cups chopped baby bok choy

1 cup fresh bean sprouts

¼ cup chopped fresh cilantro

¼ cup chopped fresh basil

1. Heat the oil in a medium saucepan, and then add the ginger and cook 30 seconds or until fragrant. Add the broth, 1 cup water, coconut aminos, and lime juice. Bring to a boil, reduce heat, cover, and simmer 10 minutes.

2. Remove from the heat, stir in the spinach, bok choy, and sprouts. Cover and let stand 5 minutes or until the bok choy is tender. Stir in the cilantro and basil.

3. Divide between 2 bowls.

Nutrition Information (per serving):

Calories 246

Carbohydrate 12g

(Fiber 3g, Sugars 5g)

Fat 19g (Saturated Fat 2g)

Protein 11g

Cholesterol 0mg

Sodium 1,147 mg

Macros: 69% Fat, 17% Protein, 14% Carbs

Net Carbs: 9g

Almond Chiller

SERVES 2 • TOTAL TIME: 5 MINUTES

1½ cups unsweetened almond milk

¼ cup almond butter

1 tablespoon hemp protein powder

6 to 9 drops liquid stevia, or more to taste

½ teaspoon vanilla extract

¼ teaspoon almond extract

1 cup ice cubes

Place all the ingredients in a blender, secure with a lid, and puree until smooth. Serve immediately.

Nutrition Information (per serving):

Calories 226
Carbohydrate 8g
(Fiber 5g, Sugars 2g)
Fat 20g (Saturated Fat 2.1g)
Protein 9g

Cholesterol 0mg
Sodium 165mg
Macros: 78% Fat, 16% Protein, 6% Carbs
Net Carbs: 3g

Mini Broccoli and "Cheese" Frittata

SERVES 1 • PREP: 5 MINUTES • BAKE: 16 MINUTES

1 tablespoon ghee, plus more for greasing ramekin

2 large eggs

⅓ cup chopped broccoli, lightly steamed

1 tablespoon finely chopped roasted red bell pepper

1 teaspoon nutritional yeast

Sea salt and black pepper

1. Preheat oven to 350°F. Grease a 6- or 8-ounce ramekin with some ghee.

2. In a medium bowl, beat the eggs. Stir in the broccoli, roasted pepper, the 1 tablespoon ghee, nutritional yeast, and a pinch each of salt and pepper.

3. Pour into the prepared ramekin. Bake for 16 to 18 minutes or until cooked through.

Nutrition Information (per serving):

Calories 273
Carbohydrate 3g
(Fiber 1g, Sugars 1g)
Fat 24g (Saturated Fat 11.5g)
Protein 13g

Cholesterol 381mg
Sodium 493mg
Macros: 78% Fat, 20% Protein, 2% Carbs
Net Carbs: 2g

Overnight Lemon-Raspberry Chia Pudding

SERVES 1 • **PREP: 5 MINUTES** • **CHILL: OVERNIGHT**

⅔ cup full-fat coconut milk

2 tablespoons hemp protein powder

1½ tablespoons chia seeds

½ teaspoon grated lemon zest

1½ teaspoons fresh lemon juice

⅛ teaspoon vanilla extract

Sea salt

Liquid stevia (optional)

¼ cup fresh raspberries

¼ cup chopped pistachios

1 tablespoon hemp seeds

1. In a 2-cup glass jar with lid or a small bowl, combine the coconut milk, protein powder, chia seeds, lemon zest and juice, vanilla, a pinch of sea salt, and a few drops of liquid stevia, if desired. Stir to combine.

2. Cover and chill overnight.

3. When ready to eat, top with raspberries, pistachios, and hemp seeds.

Nutrition Information (per serving):

Calories 404

Carbohydrate 18g

(Fiber 12g, Sugars 5g)

Fat 35g (Saturated Fat 21.5g)

Protein 16g

Cholesterol 0mg

Sodium 199mg

Macros: 78% Fat, 16% Protein, 6% Carbs

Net Carbs: 6g

Cream Cheese with Salmon Wrap-Ups

SERVES 2 • TOTAL TIME: 10 MINUTES

4 ounces vegan cream cheese

2 tablespoons finely chopped red onion

2 teaspoons small capers

½ teaspoon dried oregano

1 cup chopped spinach

2 coconut wraps

¼ cup thinly sliced cucumber

4 ounces smoked salmon

2 hard-boiled eggs, peeled and chopped

1. Stir together the cream cheese, onion, capers, and oregano in a medium bowl. Add the spinach and stir until well blended.

2. Top each wrap with equal amounts of the cream cheese mixture and spread evenly. Top with equal amounts of the cucumber, salmon, and egg. Roll up or serve open-faced with knife and fork.

Nutrition Information (per serving):

Calories 415

Carbohydrate 17g

(Fiber 4g, Sugars 5g)

Fat 29g (Saturated Fat 13.1g)

Protein 25g

Cholesterol 199mg

Sodium 769mg

Macros: 63% Fat, 24% Protein, 13% Carbs

Net Carbs: 13g

Kale Caesar Salad with Eggs

SERVES 1 • TOTAL TIME: 10 MINUTES

2 cups torn kale

1½ tablespoons extra-virgin olive oil, divided

Sea salt

1 teaspoon finely chopped anchovies

1 small garlic clove, minced

1½ teaspoons fresh lemon juice

1 teaspoon nutritional yeast

½ teaspoon Dijon mustard

2 tablespoons pine nuts, toasted

2 tablespoons hemp seeds

2 large hard-boiled eggs, peeled and cut into quarters

1. In a medium bowl, massage the kale with 1½ teaspoons of the olive oil and a pinch of salt until the kale starts to get tender, 1 to 2 minutes; set aside.

2. Mash the anchovies and garlic into a paste on a cutting board. Transfer to another medium bowl. Add the lemon juice, nutritional yeast, and mustard. Whisk in the remaining 1 tablespoon olive oil. Add the massaged kale leaves and toss to coat. Transfer to a serving plate and sprinkle with the pine nuts and hemp seeds. Top with the eggs.

Nutrition Information (per serving):

Calories 469

Carbohydrate 8g

(Fiber 3g, Sugars 2g)

Fat 44g (Saturated Fat 4.5g)

Protein 14g

Cholesterol 10mg

Sodium 636mg

Macros: 84% Fat, 12% Protein, 4% Carbs

Net Carbs: 5g

Carrot and Lentil Salad

SERVES 2 • PREP: 5 MINUTES • COOK: 22 MINUTES

¼ cup dried lentils

¾ cup chopped red bell pepper

½ cup matchstick carrots

1 teaspoon grated fresh ginger

1 garlic clove, minced

⅛ to ¼ teaspoon crushed red pepper flakes

2 tablespoon extra-virgin olive oil

1 tablespoon cider vinegar

½ teaspoon kosher salt

1 tablespoon avocado oil

⅓ cup slivered almonds

½ teaspoon caraway seeds

½ teaspoon dried fennel seeds

¼ teaspoon ground cumin

½ cup chopped fresh cilantro

1. Cook the lentils according to package directions or until they are cooked but still retain a bite. Place in a fine mesh sieve and run under cold water to stop the cooking process and cool quickly. Place the lentils in a medium bowl with the bell pepper, carrots, ginger, garlic, pepper flakes, olive oil, vinegar, and salt, and set aside.

2. In a large skillet, heat the avocado oil over medium heat and add the almonds, caraway seeds, fennel seeds, and cumin. Cook until the seeds begin to pop, about 2 minutes, stirring frequently. Stir into the lentil mixture with the cilantro.

Nutrition Information (per serving):

Calories 388

Carbohydrate 26g

(Fiber 7g, Sugars 5g)

Fat 30g (Saturated Fat 3.6g)

Protein 11g

Cholesterol 0mg

Sodium 508mg

Macros: 69% Fat, 11% Protein, 20% Carbs

Net Carbs: 19g

Lemon-Caper Tuna Salad with Cucumber "Chips"

SERVES 1 • TOTAL TIME: 10 MINUTES

1 (5-ounce) can wild albacore tuna, drained

2 tablespoons chopped fresh parsley

2 tablespoons pine nuts, toasted

1 tablespoon capers

1 tablespoon minced shallot

2 tablespoons extra-virgin olive oil

½ teaspoon grated lemon zest

1 tablespoon fresh lemon juice

½ teaspoon Dijon mustard

Kosher salt and black pepper

½ cup cucumber slices

In a medium bowl, combine the tuna, parsley, pine nuts, capers, and shallot. In a small bowl, whisk together the olive oil, lemon zest and juice, mustard, and a pinch each of salt and pepper. Drizzle over tuna mixture and toss to combine. Serve with cucumber slices.

Nutrition Information (per serving):

Calories 547

Carbohydrate 6g

(Fiber 2g, Sugars 2g)

Fat 44g (Saturated Fat 6g)

Protein 35g

Cholesterol 30mg

Sodium 628mg

Macros: 72% Fat, 25% Protein, 3% Carbs

Net Carbs: 4g

Fresh Dill, Shrimp, and Penne Salad

SERVES 2 • **PREP: 6 MINUTES** • **COOK: 7 MINUTES**

¾ cup uncooked chickpea penne pasta

6 ounces peeled raw shrimp

½ cup frozen green peas

½ cup chopped cucumber

½ cup chopped celery

⅓ cup chopped red onion

2 to 3 tablespoons chopped fresh dill

¼ cup extra-virgin olive oil

3 to 4 tablespoons fresh lemon juice, to taste

2 garlic cloves, minced

1 teaspoon Dijon mustard

Salt and black pepper

2 ounces vegan feta cheese, crumbled

1. Cook the pasta according to package directions. Add the shrimp 4 minutes before the end of cooking time. Drain in a colander. Add the frozen peas to the pasta mixture in the colander and run under cold water to cool; this will stop the cooking process and thaw the peas quickly. Drain well, shaking off excess liquid.

2. Meanwhile, in a medium bowl, combine the cucumber, celery, red onion, dill, olive oil, lemon juice, garlic, and mustard. Toss until well blended.

3. Add the drained pasta mixture and toss until well coated. Season with salt and pepper to taste.

4. Divide between 2 plates and sprinkle cheese evenly over all.

Nutrition Information (per serving):

Calories 541

Carbohydrate 32g

(Fiber 5g, Sugars 5g)

Fat 39g (Saturated Fat 11.2g)

Protein 21g

Cholesterol 107mg

Sodium 801mg

Macros: 65% Fat, 15% Protein, 20% Carbs

Net Carbs: 27g

Middle Eastern Spiced Beef on Carrot Spirals

SERVES 2 • PREP: 5 MINUTES • COOK: 20 MINUTES

- 3 tablespoons coconut oil, divided
- ¼ cup chopped pecans
- 8 ounces 93% lean grass-fed ground sirloin
- ¾ cup chopped red bell pepper
- ½ cup chopped onion
- ½ teaspoon ground cinnamon
- ¼ teaspoon ground cumin
- ⅛ teaspoon ground allspice
- ½ teaspoon kosher salt
- Black pepper
- ¼ cup chopped fresh mint, divided
- 2 to 4 drops liquid stevia (optional)
- 1 (12-ounce) package frozen carrot veggie spirals
- ¼ cup unsweetened plain vegan yogurt

1. In a medium skillet, heat 1 tablespoon of oil over medium-high heat, tilting skillet to lightly coat the bottom. Add the pecans and cook for 2 to 3 minutes or until they are fragrant and beginning to lightly brown, stirring frequently. Set aside on a plate.

2. In the same skillet, heat 1 tablespoon of oil, add the beef, and cook for 2 minutes, stirring constantly. Stir in the bell pepper and onion and cook for 8 minutes or until the onion is tender, stirring frequently. Stir in the pecans, cinnamon, cumin, allspice, salt, and black pepper to taste. Cook for 1 minute, stirring constantly. Remove from heat, stir in 3 tablespoons of the mint, 2 tablespoons water, and stevia, if desired. Cover to keep warm.

3. Meanwhile, cook the veggie spirals according to package directions. Drain well and spoon the remaining 1 tablespoon oil over the spirals. Divide the spirals between 2 plates. Spoon the beef mixture over the spirals and top with yogurt and the remaining 1 tablespoon of mint.

Nutrition Information (per serving):

Calories 551	Cholesterol 73mg
Carbohydrate 26g	Sodium 680mg
(Fiber 10g, Sugars 13g)	**Macros:** 67% Fat, 21% Protein,
Fat 41g (Saturated Fat 22g)	12% Carbs
Protein 29g	**Net Carbs:** 16g

Lox Deviled Eggs with Spinach

SERVES 1 • TOTAL TIME: 10 MINUTES

2 hard-boiled eggs, peeled and cut in half

1½ tablespoons avocado oil mayonnaise

2 teaspoons chopped fresh dill

1 teaspoon Dijon mustard

1 teaspoon chopped capers

Sea salt and black pepper

2 ounces lox or smoked salmon, torn into small pieces

1½ cups baby spinach

1 tablespoon extra-virgin olive oil

1 tablespoon fresh lemon juice

1. Scoop egg yolks into a small bowl. Add mayonnaise, dill, mustard, capers, and a pinch each of salt and pepper. Mash with a fork. Spoon back into egg whites. Top with the salmon pieces.

2. In a medium bowl, toss together the spinach, olive oil, and lemon juice. Season with a pinch each of salt and black pepper.

3. Serve eggs with spinach salad.

Nutrition Information (per serving):

Calories 476

Carbohydrate 4g

(Fiber 2g, Sugars 0g)

Fat 41g (Saturated Fat 6.5g)

Protein 25g

Cholesterol 386mg

Sodium 1028mg

Macros: 78% Fat, 21% Protein, 2% Carbs

Net Carbs: 2g

Beef Roll Ups

SERVES 2 • PREP: 6 MINUTES • COOK: 8 MINUTES

1 tablespoon avocado oil

8 ounces 93% lean grass-fed ground sirloin

1 poblano chile pepper, stemmed, seeded, and chopped

¼ cup chopped onion

1 teaspoon smoked paprika

½ teaspoon ground cumin

¼ teaspoon kosher salt

2 large eggs, well beaten (optional)

¼ cup unsweetened plain vegan yogurt

2 teaspoons fresh lime juice

1 tablespoon finely chopped fresh cilantro

2 sacha inchi wraps, warmed, such as Keto Thin Traditional Wraps by Julian Bakery

1 avocado, pitted, peeled, and sliced

2 teaspoons hot sauce, or to taste

1. In a medium skillet, heat avocado oil over medium heat until hot. Add beef and cook for 2 minutes. Add the poblano pepper, onion, paprika, cumin, and salt; cook 6 minutes, or until vegetables are tender, stirring occasionally. If desired, stir in the eggs and cook 1 minute or until set, stirring occasionally.

2. Meanwhile, combine the yogurt, lime juice, and cilantro in a small bowl and set aside.

3. Put each wrap on a plate and place avocado slices down the center of each wrap. Spoon the beef mixture on top of the avocado, drizzle hot sauce over the beef, spoon the yogurt mixture over all, and roll up.

Nutrition Information (per serving):

Version without eggs:
Calories 473
Carbohydrate 20g
(Fiber 13g, Sugars 4g)
Fat 36g (Saturated Fat 6.9g)
Protein 30g
Cholesterol 73mg
Sodium 530mg
Macros: 68% Fat, 26% Protein, 6% Carbs
Net Carbs: 7g

Version with eggs:
Calories 542
Carbohydrate 21g
(Fiber 13g, Sugars 4g)
Fat 41g (Saturated Fat 8.5g)
Protein 37g
Cholesterol 259mg
Sodium 601mg
Macros: 67% Fat, 27% Protein, 6% Carbs
Net Carbs: 8g

Keto Cinnamon Granola Cereal

SERVES 1 • COOK: 5 MINUTES

¼ cup chopped almonds

2 tablespoons pumpkin seeds (pepitas)

2 tablespoons sunflower seeds

1 tablespoon avocado oil

½ teaspoon ground cinnamon

Liquid stevia (optional)

⅓ cup unsweetened almond milk

1. In a large skillet, combine almonds, pumpkin seeds, sunflower seeds, and avocado oil. Cook over medium heat 4 to 5 minutes or until golden and fragrant, stirring frequently. Stir in the cinnamon and remove from heat. If desired, stir in a few drops of liquid stevia.

2. Serve with almond milk.

Nutrition Information (per serving):

Calories 554

Carbohydrate 14g

(Fiber 7g, Sugars 2g)

Fat 50g (Saturated Fat 5.5g)

Protein 19g

Cholesterol 0mg

Sodium 210mg

Macros: 81% Fat, 14% Protein, 5% Carbs

Net Carbs: 7g

Tropical Yogurt Bowl

SERVES 1 • TOTAL TIME: 5 MINUTES

½ cup plain Greek-style vegan yogurt

Liquid stevia (optional)

¼ cup peeled and coarsely chopped kiwi

1 tablespoon unsweetened dried coconut flakes, toasted

1 tablespoon hemp seeds

1 tablespoon chopped cashews, toasted

Place the yogurt in a serving bowl. If desired, stir in a few drops of stevia. Top with kiwi, coconut flakes, hemp seeds, and cashews.

Nutrition Information (per serving):

Calories 310

Carbohydrate 16g

(Fiber 3g, Sugars 6g)

Fat 22g (Saturated Fat 3.5g)

Protein 15g

Cholesterol 0mg

Sodium 156mg

Macros: 64% Fat, 20% Protein, 16% Carbs

Net Carbs: 13g

Crispy Trout with Buttery Shallots and Arugula

SERVES 2 • PREP: 8 MINUTES • COOK: 7 MINUTES

2 tablespoons ghee, divided

¼ cup finely minced shallots

1 tablespoon fresh lemon juice

¼ cup almond flour

2 skin-on trout fillets (6 ounces each), rinsed and patted dry

1 tablespoon avocado oil

Pinch of cayenne pepper

Kosher salt and black pepper

2 cups arugula

½ lemon

2 tablespoons chopped fresh parsley

1. Heat a large nonstick skillet over medium-high heat and add 1 tablespoon of ghee. When the ghee has melted, add the shallots and cook until beginning to lightly brown. Remove from heat, stir in the 1 tablespoon of lemon juice, and set aside in small bowl.

2. Place the flour in a large, flat dish. Coat fillets on both sides, shaking off any excess flour.

3. In the same skillet, heat the oil and the remaining 1 tablespoon of ghee over medium-high heat. When the ghee has melted, reduce the heat to medium, add the fish and cook for 2 minutes. Carefully turn the fillets over, and sprinkle with cayenne, ¼ teaspoon of salt, and black pepper to taste. Cook 2 minutes or until the fish flakes easily with a fork. Remove the skillet from the heat.

4. Divide the arugula between 2 plates and squeeze the lemon half evenly over the arugula. Sprinkle with salt and pepper to taste. Place the fish on top of the arugula. Whisk the shallot mixture, spoon over the fish, and sprinkle with parsley.

Nutrition Information (per serving):

Calories 455

Carbohydrate 7g

(Fiber 2g, Sugars 3g)

Fat 34g (Saturated Fat 11.3g)

Protein 32g

Cholesterol 105mg

Sodium 326mg

Macros: 68% Fat, 28% Protein, 4% Carbs

Net Carbs: 5g

Mushroom-Spinach Mini Quiche

SERVES: 1 • PREP: 5 MINUTES • COOK: 6 MINUTES • BAKE: 16 MINUTES

1 tablespoon ghee plus additional for greasing ramekin

½ cup sliced mushrooms

2 cups baby spinach

2 large eggs, beaten

Sea salt and black pepper

1-ounce slice vegan mozzarella cheese

1. Preheat the oven to 350°F. Grease a 6- to 8-ounce ramekin with some ghee.

2. In a small skillet, heat the 1 tablespoon ghee over medium heat. When the ghee has melted, add the mushrooms and cook until wilted, 5 to 6 minutes. Stir in the spinach and cook 1 minute or just until wilted. Remove from heat.

3. In a medium bowl, combine the beaten eggs with the mushroom mixture and a pinch each of salt and pepper. Pour into prepared ramekin. Top with cheese. Bake for 16 to 18 minutes or until cooked through.

Nutrition Information (per serving):

Calories 412

Carbohydrate 10g

(Fiber 3g, Sugars 2g)

Fat 35g (Saturated Fat 19g)

Protein 18g

Cholesterol 390mg

Sodium 426mg

Macros: 76% Fat, 17% Protein, 7% Carbs

Net Carbs: 7g

Zucchini-Asparagus Hash

SERVES 1 • PREP: 5 MINUTES • COOK: 5 MINUTES

2 tablespoons ghee, divided

½ cup chopped zucchini

½ cup chopped asparagus

Sea salt and black pepper

2 large eggs

1 teaspoon nutritional yeast

1. In a small skillet, heat 1 tablespoon of the ghee over medium-high heat. When the ghee has melted, add the zucchini and asparagus and cook for 3 to 4 minutes, or until tender crisp. Season with a pinch each of salt and pepper. Add the remaining 1 tablespoon ghee to the pan. Crack the eggs over the vegetables. Sprinkle with the nutritional yeast and another pinch each of salt and pepper.

2. Cover and cook, undisturbed, 2 minutes or until eggs reach desired doneness.

Nutrition Information (per serving):

Calories 416

Carbohydrate 3g

(Fiber 1g, Sugars 1g)

Fat 38g (Saturated Fat 20g)

Protein 15g

Cholesterol 410mg

Sodium 276mg

Macros: 83% Fat, 14% Protein, 3% Carbs

Net Carbs: 2g

Avocado + Grapefruit with Coconut Topping

SERVES 2 • TOTAL TIME: 10 MINUTES

- ¼ cup full-fat coconut milk
- 1 tablespoon fresh lime juice
- ½ teaspoon grated fresh ginger
- 2 to 4 drops liquid stevia, or to taste
- 1 avocado, pitted, peeled, and sliced
- 1 pink grapefruit, cut into sections
- ⅓ cup pistachio nuts, coarsely chopped
- 2 tablespoons unsweetened dried coconut flakes

1. In a small bowl, combine the coconut milk, lime juice, ginger, and stevia. Stir until well blended.

2. Divide the avocado and grapefruit sections between 2 plates. Spoon the coconut milk mixture evenly over each serving and sprinkle with the pistachios and coconut.

Nutrition Information (per serving):

Calories 409
Carbohydrate 32g
(Fiber 11g, Sugars 14g)
Fat 33g (Saturated Fat 11g)
Protein 8g

Cholesterol 0mg
Sodium 13mg
Macros: 72% Fat, 8% Protein, 20% Carbs
Net Carbs: 21

Natto-Rice Bowls

SERVES 2 • TOTAL TIME: 10 MINUTES (IF USING COOKED RICE);
25 MINUTES (IF USING UNCOOKED RICE AND COOKING IT)

- 2 (50-gram) packets natto (fermented soybeans)
- ½ teaspoon Dijon mustard (or hot Japanese yellow mustard)
- ¼ teaspoon wasabi paste (optional)
- ½ cup hot cooked white rice, preferably short grain
- 2 teaspoons coconut aminos, or to taste
- ¼ cup finely chopped green onions
- 2 avocados, pitted, peeled, and chopped

1. In a small bowl, combine the natto with the mustard and wasabi paste, if using. Mix vigorously until well blended.

2. Divide rice between 2 bowls and top with equal amounts of the natto mixture, coconut aminos, green onions, and avocado. Serve immediately.

Quick Tip: Store cooked rice in the freezer to have on hand. Reheat it in the microwave or in a small amount of boiling water.

Nutrition Information (per serving):

Calories 438
Carbohydrate 38g
(Fiber 17g, Sugars 4g)
Fat 34g (Saturated Fat 5.3g)
Protein 13g

Cholesterol 0mg
Sodium 410mg
Macros: 69% Fat, 12% Protein, 19% Carbs
Net Carbs: 21g

Spicy Chicken Patties with Pineapple

SERVES 2 • PREP: 8 MINUTES • COOK: 6 MINUTES

8 ounces ground chicken

¼ cup finely chopped red bell pepper

2 tablespoons finely chopped red onion

2 tablespoons chopped fresh mint

2 teaspoons grated fresh ginger

⅛ teaspoon kosher salt

⅛ teaspoon black pepper

2 tablespoons coconut oil

1 cup fresh pineapple chunks, about 1-inch pieces

⅛ teaspoon crushed red pepper flakes (optional)

1. In a medium bowl, combine chicken, bell pepper, onion, mint, ginger, salt, and black pepper. Shape into 4 small patties, about 2 to 2½ inches in diameter.

2. Heat the coconut oil in a large skillet over medium heat, tilting skillet to lightly coat the bottom. When hot, add the patties and the pineapple chunks in a single layer. Sprinkle with pepper flakes, if desired. Cook 3 minutes on one side. Turn the patties and pineapple and cook for 3 to 4 minutes or until patties are no longer pink in the center.

3. Divide patties between 2 plates and place pineapple alongside.

Nutrition Information (per serving):

Calories 337

Carbohydrate 14g

(Fiber 2g, Sugars 9g)

Fat 23g (Saturated Fat 14g)

Protein 21g

Cholesterol 98mg

Sodium 217mg

Macros: 61% Fat, 25% Protein, 14% Carbs

Net Carbs: 12g

Grilled Halibut on Tzatziki Greens

SERVES 2 • PREP: 10 MINUTES • COOK: 8 MINUTES

Sauce

- ½ cup unsweetened plain vegan yogurt
- 1 tablespoon extra-virgin olive oil
- 2 teaspoons dried dill
- 1 garlic clove, minced
- ¼ teaspoon kosher salt

Salad

- 2 halibut steaks (4 ounces each), rinsed and patted dry
- 2 tablespoons olive or avocado oil, divided
- ⅛ teaspoon kosher salt
- Black pepper to taste
- 3 cups torn endive leaves
- 1 cup thinly sliced cucumber
- ¼ cup thinly sliced radishes
- 3 tablespoons chopped fresh mint, divided
- 1 lemon, halved

1. Preheat grill or grill pan to medium-high heat.

2. To make the sauce: combine the yogurt, olive oil, 1½ tablespoons water, dill, garlic, and salt in a small bowl and set aside.

3. Brush both sides of the fish with 1 tablespoon of oil and sprinkle with the salt and black pepper. Place on the grill or in the grill pan and cook 4 to 5 minutes on each side or until the fish flakes easily with a fork. Break into smaller pieces.

4. To make the salad: Divide the endive, cucumber, radishes, and 2 tablespoons of mint between 2 plates. Top with equal amounts of the sauce and flaked fish. Drizzle remaining 1 tablespoon of oil over all and sprinkle with remaining 1 tablespoon of mint. Squeeze lemon halves over all.

Nutrition Information (per serving):

Calories 366
Carbohydrate 10g
(Fiber 4g, Sugars 2g)
Fat 27g (Saturated Fat 3.7g)
Protein 25g

Cholesterol 59mg
Sodium 467mg
Macros: 66% Fat, 27% Protein, 7% Carbs
Net Carbs: 6g

Chilled Sweet Pea + Avocado Soup

SERVES 2 • TOTAL TIME: 10 MINUTES

1 avocado

1 cup frozen green peas

1 cup unsweetened almond milk

¾ cup full-fat coconut milk

½ cup chopped fresh cilantro

½ cup unsweetened plain vegan yogurt, divided

2 tablespoons fresh lemon juice

1 teaspoon hot sauce

Kosher salt and black pepper

1. Cut the avocado in half and remove the pit. Using a spoon, scoop out the "meat" of the avocado and place in a blender with the peas, almond milk, coconut milk, cilantro, ¼ cup of the yogurt, lemon juice, hot sauce, and ¼ teaspoon salt. Secure with lid and puree until smooth. Season with additional salt and pepper to taste.

2. Divide between 2 bowls and top with remaining ¼ cup yogurt.

Nutrition Information (per serving):

Calories 444

Carbohydrate 27g

(Fiber 13g, Sugars 5g)

Fat 39g (Saturated Fat 18.6g)

Protein 10g

Cholesterol 4mg

Sodium 468mg

Macros: 78% Fat, 9% Protein, 13% Carbs

Net Carbs: 14g

Smashed Bean Wraps

SERVES 2 • TOTAL TIME: 15 MINUTES

1 cup canned organic pinto beans, rinsed and drained

3 tablespoons extra-virgin olive oil, divided

¼ teaspoon ground chipotle

½ teaspoon kosher salt, divided

2 coconut wraps

1 avocado, pitted, peeled, and sliced

1 cup shredded red cabbage

¼ cup chopped radishes

¼ cup chopped fresh cilantro or finely chopped green onions

1 tablespoon fresh lime juice

⅛ teaspoon black pepper

¼ cup unsweetened plain vegan yogurt

1. In a medium bowl, roughly mash the beans with 2 tablespoons of olive oil, the ground chipotle, and ¼ teaspoon salt until well blended. Place the coconut wraps on separate plates and spread each one with equal amounts of the bean mixture. Top with avocado slices.

2. In the same bowl that you used for the beans, combine the cabbage, radishes, cilantro, lime juice, remaining 1 tablespoon of oil, remaining ¼ teaspoon of salt, and the black pepper. Toss until well blended.

3. Top each coconut wrap with equal amounts of the cabbage mixture. Spoon yogurt on top. Roll up or serve open-faced.

Nutrition Information (per serving):

Calories 535

Carbohydrate 38g

(Fiber 17g, Sugars 4g)

Fat 46g (Saturated Fat 12.3g)

Protein 10g

Cholesterol 0mg

Sodium 537mg

Macros: 77% Fat, 8% Protein, 15% Carbs

Net Carbs: 21g

Chicken, Cabbage, and Sunflower Seed Salad

SERVES 2 • TOTAL TIME: 15 MINUTES

Dressing

- 3 tablespoons avocado oil
- 2 tablespoons coconut aminos
- 1 tablespoon apple cider vinegar
- 6 to 9 drops liquid stevia, or to taste
- 2 teaspoons grated fresh ginger or orange zest

Salad

- 2 tablespoons hulled sunflower seeds
- 3 cups shredded green cabbage
- ¾ cup sugar snap peas, cut in half diagonally
- 1 cup cooked chopped chicken breast
- ¼ cup chopped red onion
- 1 red jalapeño, halved lengthwise, seeded, and sliced
- ¼ cup chopped fresh cilantro

1. To make the dressing: In a small bowl, whisk together the avocado oil, coconut aminos, cider vinegar, liquid stevia, and grated ginger and set aside.

2. To make the salad: Heat a medium skillet over medium-high heat. Add the sunflower seeds to the skillet and cook for 2 minutes or until beginning to lightly brown, stirring frequently. Remove from the heat.

3. In a large bowl, combine the cabbage, snap peas, chicken, onion, jalapeño, and cilantro. Pour the dressing over all and toss until well blended.

4. Divide the salad between 2 plates. Top with equal amounts of the sunflower seeds.

Nutrition Information (per serving):

Calories 395
Carbohydrate 15g
(Fiber 4g, Sugars 2g)
Fat 28g (Saturated Fat 3.6g)
Protein 26g

Cholesterol 60mg
Sodium 654mg
Macros: 63% Fat, 26% Protein, 11% Carbs
Net Carbs: 11g

Arugula-Grapefruit Salad

SERVES 1 • TOTAL TIME: 10 MINUTES

2 cups baby arugula

¼ cup fresh grapefruit sections

1 ounce vegan fresh-style mozzarella cheese, cubed

2 tablespoons pumpkin seeds (pepitas), toasted

1 tablespoon hemp seeds, toasted

2 tablespoons extra-virgin olive oil

1 tablespoon fresh lemon juice

1 teaspoon nutritional yeast

Sea salt and black pepper

1. In a medium bowl, combine the arugula, grapefruit, and cheese. Transfer to a serving plate. Sprinkle with pumpkin seeds and hemp seeds.

2. In a small bowl, whisk together the olive oil, lemon juice, nutritional yeast, and a pinch each of salt and pepper. Drizzle over the arugula mixture.

Nutrition Information (per serving):

Calories 541

Carbohydrate 17g

(Fiber 4g, Sugars 7g)

Fat 48g (Saturated Fat 10.5g)

Protein 14g

Cholesterol 0mg

Sodium 242mg

Macros: 80% Fat, 11% Protein, 10% Carbs

Net Carbs: 13g

Walnut and Chicken–Stuffed Celery

SERVES 1 • TOTAL TIME: 5 MINUTES

½ cup shredded cooked chicken breast

2 tablespoons chopped toasted walnuts

2 tablespoons avocado oil mayonnaise

1 tablespoon fresh lemon juice

1 teaspoon Dijon mustard

Kosher salt and black pepper

2 celery stalks, cut into 3-inch pieces

1 tablespoon chia seeds

1. In a medium bowl, combine the chicken, walnuts, mayonnaise, lemon juice, mustard, and a pinch each of salt and pepper.

2. Stuff celery stalks with chicken salad. Sprinkle with chia seeds.

Nutrition Information (per serving):

Calories 438

Carbohydrate 7g

(Fiber 3g, Sugars 2g)

Fat 36g (Saturated Fat 4.5g)

Protein 25g

Cholesterol 98mg

Sodium 844mg

Macros: 74% Fat, 23% Protein, 4% Carbs

Net Carbs: 4g

Chicken and Mushrooms with Balsamic-Wine Reduction

SERVES 2 • PREP: 10 MINUTES • COOK: 30 MINUTES

½ teaspoon kosher salt, divided

Black pepper to taste

2 boneless, skinless chicken breasts (4 ounces each), flattened to an even thickness

2 tablespoons olive oil, divided

3 tablespoons chopped fresh parsley, divided

4 ounces sliced baby portobello (cremini) mushrooms

1 green onion, finely chopped

⅓ cup red wine

1½ tablespoons balsamic vinegar

2 tablespoons ghee

1. Preheat oven to 400°F. Sprinkle ¼ teaspoon of the salt and black pepper over both sides of the chicken pieces.

2. Heat a medium skillet over medium-high heat. Add 1 tablespoon of the oil and tilt skillet to lightly coat the bottom. Cook the chicken on one side for 3 minutes or until lightly browned. Place the chicken, browned side up, in a 1- to 1½-quart baking dish or shallow pie pan. Sprinkle with 2 tablespoons of the parsley.

3. Add remaining 1 tablespoon oil to the skillet. Place the mushrooms and green onion in the skillet and cook over medium-high for 4 minutes or until the mushrooms begin to brown, stirring occasionally. Stir in the remaining ¼ teaspoon of salt. Spoon over the chicken.

4. Add the wine and vinegar to the skillet. Bring to a boil over medium-high heat and boil for 2 to 3 minutes or until reduced to 2 tablespoons of liquid. Remove from heat and stir in the ghee. Spoon over the mushroom mixture; sprinkle with black pepper.

5. Bake, uncovered, 20 to 22 minutes or until chicken is no longer pink in the center. Sprinkle with remaining parsley. Let stand 5 minutes to absorb flavors.

Nutrition Information (per serving):

Calories 422

Carbohydrate 9g

(Fiber 2g, Sugars 5g)

Fat 31g (Saturated Fat 11.1g)

Protein 28g

Cholesterol 105mg

Sodium 550mg

Macros: 67% Fat, 27% Protein, 6% Carbs

Net Carbs: 7g

Tarragon Beet Salad with Cream Cheese "Croutons"

SERVES 2 • PREP: 15 MINUTES • COOK: 20 MINUTES

10 ounces beets, ends trimmed

3 tablespoons olive oil, divided

1 tablespoon sesame seeds

1 tablespoon hemp seeds

4 ounces vegan cream cheese, cut into ½-inch cubes

2 cups baby spinach

2 cups torn endive leaves

½ cup thinly sliced red onion

2 tablespoons balsamic vinegar

½ teaspoon grated orange zest (optional)

1 teaspoon hot sauce

1 tablespoon coarsely chopped fresh tarragon

Kosher salt and black pepper

1. Preheat oven to 425°F. Line a baking sheet with foil.

2. Peel the beets under running water. Quickly cut into ½-inch-thick wedges and rinse fingers immediately. Dry the beets with paper towels and toss with 1 tablespoon of the oil. Place on the prepared baking sheet and roast for 10 minutes. Turn the beets over and roast for 7 to 8 minutes or until just tender when pierced with a fork. Set aside to cool on the baking sheet.

3. Meanwhile, heat a medium skillet over medium heat until hot. Add the sesame and hemp seeds and cook for 3 to 4 minutes or until lightly toasted, stirring occasionally. Place in a shallow pan and allow to cool for 1 to 2 minutes. Working in batches, add cream cheese cubes; toss until evenly coated with seed mixture.

4. In a large bowl, combine the spinach, endive, and onion. In a small bowl, whisk together the remaining 2 tablespoons of oil, the vinegar, orange zest, if using, and hot sauce. Pour over the spinach mixture and toss until well coated.

5. Divide the spinach mixture between 2 plates, top with the beets and cheese "croutons," and sprinkle with the tarragon. Season with salt and pepper.

Nutrition Information (per serving):

Calories 500
Carbohydrate 33g
(Fiber 8g, Sugars 16g)
Fat 39g (Saturated Fat 7.3g)
Protein 13g

Cholesterol 0mg
Sodium 373mg
Macros: 70% Fat, 10% Protein, 20% Carbs
Net Carbs: 25g

Spicy Veggie Scramble

SERVES 2 • PREP: 7 MINUTES • COOK: 8 MINUTES

5 eggs

¼ teaspoon ground cumin

Kosher salt and black pepper

2 tablespoons avocado oil, divided

1 medium poblano chile pepper, seeded and chopped

½ medium onion, thinly sliced

8 ounces sliced mushrooms

3 cups arugula

1 plum tomato, finely chopped

Hot sauce

1. In a medium bowl, beat eggs with cumin and salt and black pepper to taste.

2. Heat a large skillet over medium heat. Add 1 tablespoon of the oil and tilt the skillet to lightly coat the bottom. Add the poblano pepper and onion and cook for 3 minutes or until tender crisp. Add the mushrooms and cook for 4 to 5 minutes or until they start to lightly brown, stirring frequently. Season with salt and pepper to taste.

3. Divide the arugula between 2 plates. Spoon the mushroom mixture on top of the arugula.

4. In the same skillet, add the remaining 1 tablespoon of oil and tilt the skillet to lightly coat the bottom. Add the eggs and cook 1 to 2 minutes, lifting up the eggs to allow raw portions to cook to achieve a scrambled egg texture.

5. Spoon equal amounts of scrambled egg on top of the mushrooms and arugula on each plate. Top with the chopped tomato and sprinkle with hot sauce to taste.

Nutrition Information (per serving):

Calories 374

Carbohydrate 15g

(Fiber 3g, Sugars 8g)

Fat 27g (Saturated Fat 5.6g)

Protein 22g

Cholesterol 465mg

Sodium 437mg

Macros: 64% Fat, 24% Protein, 13% Carbs

Net Carbs: 12g

Buttery Sea Scallops on Garlic Snow Peas

SERVES 2 • PREP: 5 MINUTES • COOK: 10 MINUTES

12 ounces sea scallops

1½ tablespoons olive oil

1½ cups snow peas, stems trimmed

2 garlic cloves, minced

¼ teaspoon kosher salt, divided

⅛ teaspoon paprika

Black pepper

2 tablespoons ghee, divided

¼ cup finely chopped shallots

2 tablespoons chopped fresh parsley

2 lemon wedges

1. Place the scallops on several layers of paper towels and gently press to release liquid. Set aside.

2. Heat the oil over medium-high heat in a large skillet, tilting the skillet to lightly coat the bottom. Add the snow peas and cook 3 minutes or until just beginning to brown on edges, tossing gently. Add the garlic and ⅛ teaspoon of salt; cook 30 seconds, stirring constantly. Set aside on a separate plate. Cover to keep warm.

3. Season the scallops with paprika, remaining ⅛ teaspoon of salt, and black pepper to taste.

4. In the same skillet, melt 1 tablespoon of the ghee over medium heat. Add the scallops (do not crowd them) and cook 3 minutes. Turn and cook 2 additional minutes, or until opaque. Place on a separate plate.

5. Add the remaining 1 tablespoon ghee to the skillet. Cook the shallots over medium heat 3 to 4 minutes, stirring occasionally, or until just richly browned. Stir in the scallops and toss until well coated.

6. Divide the snow peas between 2 plates. Spoon the scallop mixture on top, sprinkle with parsley, and serve with lemon wedges.

Nutrition Information (per serving):

Calories 368

Carbohydrate 14g

(Fiber 2g, Sugars 4g)

Fat 26g (Saturated Fat 10.2g)

Protein 23g

Cholesterol 63mg

Sodium 914mg

Macros: 62% Fat, 25% Protein, 13% Carbs

Net Carbs: 12g

Sweet Potato + Nut Butter Stew

SERVES 2 • PREP: 10 MINUTES • COOK: 35 MINUTES

2 tablespoons coconut oil

½ cup chopped onions

1 medium sweet potato, cut into ½-inch cubes

½ (15-ounce) can organic kidney beans, rinsed and drained

¾ cup chopped tomatoes

1 cup vegetable broth

3 tablespoons almond butter

1 teaspoon ground cumin

¼ teaspoon ground cinnamon

⅛ teaspoon cayenne pepper

2 to 3 drops liquid stevia, or to taste

⅔ cup sliced almonds

¼ cup unsweetened plain vegan yogurt

2 tablespoons chopped fresh cilantro

1. Heat the oil in a medium saucepan over medium-high heat. Add the onions and cook, stirring frequently, 6 minutes or until richly browned.

2. To the saucepan, add the sweet potato, beans, tomatoes, broth, almond butter, cumin, cinnamon, and cayenne. Bring to a boil, reduce heat, cover, and simmer, stirring occasionally, for 25 to 30 minutes or until potatoes are very tender. Remove from heat and stir in the stevia.

3. Divide between 2 bowls and top with the almonds, yogurt, and cilantro.

Nutrition Information (per serving):

Calories 483

Carbohydrate 35g

(Fiber 10g, Sugars 8g)

Fat 37g (Saturated Fat 14.2g)

Protein 14g

Cholesterol 2mg

Sodium 575mg

Macros: 68% Fat, 12% Protein, 20% Carbs

Net Carbs: 25g

Tempeh-Walnut Bowls

SERVES 2 • PREP: 10 MINUTES • COOK: 8 MINUTES

8 ounces tempeh

1 tablespoon avocado oil

⅓ cup chopped walnuts

2 garlic cloves, minced

2 teaspoons ground cumin

½ teaspoon ground chipotle, divided

½ teaspoon kosher salt

¼ cup unsweetened plain vegan yogurt

2 cups shredded romaine lettuce

1 avocado, pitted, peeled, and chopped

2 green onions, finely chopped

¼ cup chopped fresh cilantro

2 lime wedges

1. Crumble tempeh by hand or place in a food processor and pulse to a coarse and crumbly consistency, being careful not to over-pulse.

2. Heat a large skillet over medium-high heat. Add the oil and tilt the skillet to coat the bottom lightly. Add the tempeh and cook 4 to 5 minutes or until beginning to brown, breaking up larger pieces while cooking. Add the walnuts, garlic, cumin, ¼ teaspoon of the ground chipotle, and the salt. Cook 3 minutes or until fragrant, stirring frequently.

3. In a small bowl, combine the yogurt and remaining ¼ teaspoon of ground chipotle.

4. To serve, divide the lettuce between two 2 bowls. Top with the tempeh mixture, the yogurt mixture, avocado, green onions, and cilantro. Serve with lime wedges.

Nutrition Information (per serving):

Calories 523

Carbohydrate 31g

(Fiber 20g, Sugars 3g)

Fat 41g (Saturated Fat 5.2g)

Protein 29g

Cholesterol 0mg

Sodium 506mg

Macros: 70% Fat, 22% Protein, 8% Carbs

Net Carbs: 11g

Caprese Zoodle Salad

SERVES 1 • PREP: 5 MINUTES

1½ cups spiralized zucchini noodles

½ cup halved grape tomatoes

1 ounce vegan fresh-style mozzarella cheese, cubed

2 tablespoons torn fresh basil

1 tablespoon toasted pine nuts

1 tablespoon hemp seeds

2 tablespoons extra-virgin olive oil

1½ teaspoons balsamic vinegar

Sea salt and black pepper

In a medium bowl, combine the zucchini noodles, tomatoes, cheese, basil, pine nuts, and hemp seeds. Transfer to a serving plate. Drizzle with the olive oil and vinegar. Season with a pinch each of salt and pepper.

Nutrition Information (per serving):

Calories 494

Carbohydrate 19g

(Fiber 3g, Sugars 7g)

Fat 46g (Saturated Fat 9g)

Protein 8g

Cholesterol 0mg

Sodium 247mg

Macros: 81% Fat, 7% Protein, 12% Carbs

Net Carbs: 16g

VT

Egg, Nut, and Cheese Bento Box

SERVES 1 • TIME: 5 MINUTES

2 hard-boiled eggs,
peeled and cut in half

¼ cup toasted almonds

¼ cup grape tomatoes

¼ cup baby carrots

2 tablespoons vegan
chive-flavored cream
cheese

6 pitted kalamata olives

In a multi-compartmental insulated lunch box, arrange the eggs, almonds, grape tomatoes, carrots, cream cheese (for dipping carrots), and olives. Keep cool until ready to eat.

Nutrition Information (per serving):

Calories 534
Carbohydrate 21g
(Fiber 7g, Sugars 5g)
Fat 43g (Saturated Fat 9.5g)
Protein 23g

Cholesterol 350mg
Sodium 589mg
Macros: 72% Fat, 18% Protein, 10% Carbs
Net Carbs: 14g

VV

Grilled Chicken Thigh

SERVES 1 • PREP: 2 MINUTES • COOK: 5 MINUTES

1 boneless, skinless
chicken thigh
(4 ounces)

1 tablespoon avocado oil

Sea salt and black
pepper

1. Preheat grill to medium heat.

2. Rub the chicken with the avocado oil. Season with a pinch each of salt and pepper.

3. Grill 5 to 6 minutes per side or until no longer pink in the center.

Nutrition Information (per serving):

Calories 261
Carbohydrate 0g
(Fiber 0g, Sugars 0g)
Fat 20g (Saturated Fat 3.5g)
Protein 19g

Cholesterol 104mg
Sodium 211mg
Macros: 70% Fat, 30% Protein, 0% Carbs
Net Carbs: 0g

Coconut Thai Shrimp

SERVES 2 • PREP: 5 MINUTES • COOK: 20 MINUTES

1 tablespoon ghee

4 ounces sliced mushrooms

1 garlic clove, minced

2 small or medium tomatoes, chopped

1½ tablespoons Thai roasted red chili paste

10 ounces raw peeled shrimp

2 teaspoons grated fresh ginger

½ cup full-fat coconut milk

⅓ cup chopped fresh cilantro, divided

Kosher salt and black pepper

2 tablespoons unsweetened dried coconut flakes

2 lime wedges

1. Heat a medium saucepan over medium-high heat and add ghee. When melted, add the mushrooms and cook for 4 minutes or until tender, stirring occasionally. Stir in the garlic and cook 30 seconds, stirring constantly. Add the tomatoes, ⅓ cup water, and chili paste. Bring to a boil, then reduce heat, cover, and simmer 10 minutes. Add the shrimp and ginger. Cover and cook 5 minutes or until the shrimp are opaque in the center.

2. Remove from heat and stir in the coconut milk and all but 2 tablespoons of the cilantro. Cover and let stand 5 minutes to absorb flavors. Season with salt and black pepper to taste.

3. Divide between 2 bowls. Top with the remaining cilantro and the coconut flakes. Serve with lime wedges.

Nutrition Information (per serving):

Calories 342

Carbohydrate 12g

(Fiber 3g, Sugars 5g)

Fat 24g (Saturated Fat 17.5g)

Protein 24g

Cholesterol 190mg

Sodium 859mg

Macros: 62% Fat, 28% Protein, 10% Carbs

Net Carbs: 9g

Dijon Chicken with Green Onion Cauliflower

SERVES 2 • **PREP: 7 MINUTES** • **COOK: 18 MINUTES**

3 tablespoons olive oil, divided

2 tablespoons no-sugar-added whole-grain mustard

½ teaspoon dried tarragon

2 large boneless, skinless chicken thighs (about 8 ounces total), flattened slightly

Black pepper to taste

1 (10-ounce) package frozen riced cauliflower

⅓ cup finely chopped green onions, divided

⅛ teaspoon kosher salt

1. In a small bowl, whisk together 2 tablespoons of the oil with the mustard and tarragon. Reserve 2 tablespoons of the mixture and set aside. Brush the remaining mustard mixture over both sides of the chicken and sprinkle with black pepper.

2. Heat a medium nonstick skillet over medium heat. Cook the chicken thighs for 6 minutes on each side or until they are no longer pink in the center.

3. Meanwhile, cook the cauliflower according to package directions.

4. Toss the cooked cauliflower with ¼ cup of the green onions, the remaining tablespoon of oil, the salt, and black pepper. Divide between 2 plates and top with the chicken.

5. In the pan used to cook the chicken, whisk in ¼ cup water and bring to a boil over medium heat. Boil for 45 to 60 seconds or until reduced to 2 tablespoons, stirring and scraping the bottom of the pan. Remove from the heat and whisk in the reserved mustard mixture until well blended. Spoon sauce evenly over the chicken and cauliflower and sprinkle with the remaining green onions.

Nutrition Information (per serving):

Calories 396

Carbohydrate 9g

(Fiber 4g, Sugars 4g)

Fat 31g (Saturated Fat 5.4g)

Protein 25g

Cholesterol 76mg

Sodium 543mg

Macros: 70% Fat, 25% Protein, 5% Carbs

Net Carbs: 5g

Deviled Egg Long-Leaf Wraps

SERVES 2 • TOTAL TIME: 15 MINUTES

4 large hard-boiled eggs, peeled and chopped

3 tablespoons avocado oil mayonnaise

2 teaspoons cider vinegar

½ teaspoon no-sugar-added whole-grain mustard

½ teaspoon kosher salt

¾ cup chopped celery

4 to 6 large romaine lettuce leaves

½ cup chopped red bell pepper

1 to 2 jalapeños, seeded and finely chopped

Black pepper to taste

1. Place the eggs in a medium bowl with the mayonnaise, vinegar, mustard, and salt. Stir until well blended. Stir in the celery.

2. Place lettuce leaves on a plate and spoon equal amounts of the bell pepper on each romaine leaf. Top with the egg mixture. Sprinkle evenly with the jalapeños and black pepper. Fold the long sides together to resemble a hot dog bun.

Nutrition Information (per serving):

Calories 335

Carbohydrate 10g

(Fiber 4g, Sugars 5g)

Fat 28g (Saturated Fat 5.5g)

Protein 15g

Cholesterol 372mg

Sodium 693mg

Macros: 76% Fat, 17% Protein, 7% Carbs

Net Carbs: 6g

(V)

Cauliflower "Tabbouleh"

SERVES 2 • PREP: 15 MINUTES • COOK: 1 MINUTE

1½ cups freshly riced
   cauliflower

 1 small garlic clove,
   minced

¼ cup grape tomatoes,
   halved

¼ cup thinly sliced
   cucumber

¼ cup pitted kalamata
   olives

¼ cup toasted pine nuts

 2 tablespoons chopped
   fresh mint

 2 tablespoons chopped
   fresh parsley

½ teaspoon grated lemon
   zest

 2 tablespoons fresh
   lemon juice

 1 tablespoon extra-virgin
   olive oil

 1 teaspoon red wine
   vinegar

   Sea salt and black
   pepper

In a medium microwave-safe bowl, microwave riced cauliflower and garlic on high for 1 minute or until tender crisp. Stir in the tomatoes, cucumber, olives, pine nuts, mint, parsley, lemon zest and juice, olive oil, vinegar, and a pinch each of salt and pepper.

Nutrition Information (per serving):

Calories 490

Carbohydrate 22g

(Fiber 6g, Sugars 6g)

Fat 43g (Saturated Fat 3.5g)

Protein 9g

Cholesterol 0mg

Sodium 476mg

Macros: 80% Fat, 7% Protein,
13% Carbs

Net Carbs: 16g

Beef Patties, Sugar Snaps, and Horseradish Aioli

SERVES 2 • PREP: 8 MINUTES • COOK: 18 MINUTES

3 tablespoons avocado oil mayonnaise, divided

1 teaspoon prepared horseradish

1 garlic clove, minced, divided

¼ teaspoon fresh or dried rosemary, chopped

2½ tablespoons avocado oil, divided

½ cup chopped onion

1½ cups sugar snap peas

½ teaspoon kosher salt, divided

8 ounces 93% lean grass-fed ground sirloin

¼ teaspoon black pepper

1. To make the aioli: In a small bowl, combine 2 tablespoons of the mayonnaise, the horseradish, half of the garlic, and ¼ teaspoon rosemary. Set aside.

2. In a medium skillet, heat 1 tablespoon of the oil over medium-high heat. Add the onion and cook 6 to 8 minutes, stirring occasionally, until browned. Add the remaining garlic and cook for 15 seconds, stirring constantly. Remove from heat; place in a medium bowl and let stand 5 minutes to cool slightly.

3. Meanwhile, heat the same skillet over medium-high heat. When hot, add the sugar snaps and lightly coat them with ½ tablespoon of the oil. Cook, stirring occasionally, for 3 minutes. Sprinkle with ¼ teaspoon of the salt and set aside.

4. To the bowl with the onions, add the beef, remaining 1 tablespoon mayonnaise, black pepper, and remaining ¼ teaspoon salt; stir just until combined. Gently shape the mixture into 2 (⅓-inch-thick) patties. Heat the remaining tablespoon of oil in the skillet over medium-high heat. Add the patties; cook 4 minutes on each side.

5. Serve the beef patties and sugar snaps with aioli.

Nutrition Information (per serving):

Calories 422

Carbohydrate 8g

(Fiber 2g, Sugars 3g)

Fat 33g (Saturated Fat 6.4g)

Protein 26g

Cholesterol 71mg

Sodium 569mg

Macros: 71% Fat, 24% Protein, 5% Carbs

Net Carbs: 6g

Creamy Mustard and Egg Chop Salad

SERVES 2 • TOTAL TIME: 10 MINUTES

- 2 cups chopped romaine
- 1 cup chopped kale
- 1 cup chopped cucumber
- ½ cup frozen green peas, thawed
- ¼ cup chopped red onion
- ¼ cup avocado oil mayonnaise
- 1 tablespoon fresh lemon juice
- 1 garlic clove, minced
- 2 teaspoons no-sugar-added whole-grain mustard
- ½ teaspoon kosher salt
- 4 hard-boiled eggs, peeled and cut into wedges
- 2 radishes, thinly sliced
- Black pepper to taste

1. In a large bowl, combine the romaine, kale, cucumber, peas, and onion.

2. In a small bowl, stir together the mayonnaise, lemon juice, garlic, mustard, and salt. Add to the romaine mixture and toss until well blended. Top with the eggs, radishes, and black pepper.

Nutrition Information (per serving):

Calories 421
Carbohydrate 16g
(Fiber 5g, Sugars 5g)
Fat 34g (Saturated Fat 6.2g)
Protein 17g

Cholesterol 372mg
Sodium 793mg
Macros: 73% Fat, 16% Protein, 11% Carbs
Net Carbs: 11g

Curried Tuna Salad Wraps

SERVES 2 • TOTAL TIME: 15 MINUTES

2 (5-ounce) cans albacore tuna in water

1 hard-boiled egg, peeled and chopped

⅓ cup avocado oil mayonnaise

2 teaspoons curry powder

½ teaspoon kosher salt

6 to 9 drops liquid stevia, or to taste

1 (8-ounce) can sliced water chestnuts, drained and chopped

½ cup finely chopped red bell pepper

12 Bibb lettuce leaves

1 medium green onion, finely chopped

1. Drain the water from the tuna.

2. In a medium bowl, combine the drained tuna, egg, mayonnaise, curry powder, salt, and stevia. Stir until well blended. Stir in the water chestnuts and bell pepper.

3. Stack the lettuce leaves in 6 stacks of 2 leaves each. Spoon equal amounts of the tuna mixture onto each stack and top with green onion.

Nutrition Information (per serving):

Calories 493

Carbohydrate 13g

(Fiber 3g, Sugars 4g)

Fat 37g (Saturated Fat 4.8g)

Protein 31g

Cholesterol 144mg

Sodium 708mg

Macros: 67% Fat, 25% Protein, 8% Carbs

Net Carbs: 10g

Minted Chickpea Salad

SERVES 2 • TOTAL TIME: 10 MINUTES

1 cup canned organic chickpeas, rinsed and drained

¾ cup chopped cucumber

¼ cup finely chopped red onion

½ teaspoon grated lemon zest

2 to 3 tablespoons fresh lemon juice

¾ cup chopped fresh mint

½ cup chopped fresh parsley

3 tablespoons extra-virgin olive oil

1 tablespoon spirulina powder

¼ teaspoon ground allspice

½ teaspoon kosher salt

⅔ cup slivered almonds

1 ounce vegan mozzarella cheese, chopped

1. In a medium bowl, combine chickpeas, cucumber, onion, lemon zest and juice, mint, parsley, olive oil, spirulina, allspice, salt, almonds, and cheese. Toss until well blended.

2. Divide between 2 plates.

Nutrition Information (per serving):

Calories 545

Carbohydrate 40g

(Fiber 12g, Sugars 4g)

Fat 40g (Saturated Fat 6.7g)

Protein 18g

Cholesterol 0mg

Sodium 630mg

Macros: 67% Fat, 13% Protein, 20% Carbs

Net Carbs: 28g

Lentil Rotini and Asparagus Salad

SERVES 2 • PREP: 6 MINUTES • COOK: 10 MINUTES

¾ cup uncooked lentil rotini

1 cup asparagus, broken into 2-inch pieces

½ cup grape tomatoes, halved

12 pitted kalamata olives, halved

¼ cup extra-virgin olive oil

2 teaspoons grated lemon zest

2 tablespoons fresh lemon juice

1 garlic clove, minced

¼ cup chopped fresh basil

½ teaspoon fresh or dried rosemary, chopped

Kosher salt and black pepper

1. Cook the rotini according to package directions. Add in the asparagus for the last 2 minutes of cooking time. Immediately drain in a colander and run under cold water to cool quickly and stop the cooking process. Drain well.

2. In a medium bowl, combine the drained pasta mixture with the tomatoes, olives, olive oil, lemon zest and juice, garlic, basil, and rosemary. Add salt and black pepper to taste.

3. Divide between 2 plates.

Nutrition Information (per serving):

Calories 437

Carbohydrate 25g

(Fiber 5g, Sugars 3g)

Fat 35g (Saturated Fat 4.7g)

Protein 10g

Cholesterol 0mg

Sodium 636mg

Macros: 72% Fat, 9% Protein, 19% Carbs

Net Carbs: 20g

Kidney Bean and Egg Salad

SERVES 2 • **TOTAL TIME: 15 MINUTES**

⅓ cup avocado oil mayonnaise

2 teaspoons cider vinegar

2 to 4 drops liquid stevia, or to taste

¼ teaspoon Kosher salt, plus more to taste

1 (15-ounce) can organic kidney beans, rinsed and drained

1 cup chopped green bell pepper

½ cup chopped red bell pepper

1 cup chopped celery

⅓ cup chopped red onion

2 hard-boiled eggs, peeled and chopped

1 medium cucumber, cut into eighths lengthwise, then cut in half

Black pepper

1. In a medium bowl, combine the mayonnaise, vinegar, stevia, and salt. Add the beans, green and red bell peppers, celery, and onion. Stir until well coated. Add the eggs and stir gently.

2. Divide the bean mixture between 2 plates and place the cucumber spears alongside. Sprinkle lightly with salt and pepper to taste.

Nutrition Information (per serving):

Calories 498
Carbohydrate 33g
(Fiber 10g, Sugars 9g)
Fat 38g (Saturated Fat 5.8g)
Protein 16g

Cholesterol 186mg
Sodium 778mg
Macros: 69% Fat, 13% Protein, 18% Carbs
Net Carbs: 23g

Tikka Masala–Style Chickpea Bowls

SERVES 4 • PREP: 10 MINUTES • COOK: 40 MINUTES

2 tablespoons ghee, divided

1 cup chopped onion

1½ cups sliced carrots, fresh or frozen

1 (8-ounce) can tomato sauce

2 teaspoons curry powder

1 (13.5-ounce) can full-fat coconut milk

1 (15-ounce) can organic chickpeas, rinsed and drained

2 teaspoons grated fresh ginger

2 teaspoons hot sauce

¼ teaspoon Kosher salt, plus more to taste

½ cup chopped fresh cilantro, divided

2 to 4 drops liquid stevia, or to taste

⅔ cup cooked white rice (or long grain white rice)

½ cup peanuts, chopped

¼ cup hemp seeds

1. Heat 1 tablespoon of the ghee in a large nonstick skillet over medium-high heat. When melted, tilt the skillet to lightly coat the bottom. Add the onion and cook for 6 minutes or until beginning to lightly brown on the edges, stirring occasionally. Add the carrots, tomato sauce, ½ cup water, and the curry powder. Bring to a boil over medium-high heat, reduce heat to low, cover, and cook, stirring occasionally, for 25 minutes or until the carrots are very tender.

2. Stir the coconut milk, chickpeas, ginger, hot sauce, and salt into the carrot mixture and cook 5 minutes. Remove from the heat, stir in the remaining 1 tablespoon ghee, all but 2 tablespoons of the cilantro, and the stevia. Cover and let stand for 30 minutes to blend the flavors.

3. Immediately before serving, in a small microwave-safe bowl, combine the rice, peanuts, hemp seeds, remaining 2 tablespoons of cilantro, and salt to taste. Cover and microwave on high setting for 1 minute or until heated through.

4. Spoon equal amounts of the chickpea mixture into each of 4 shallow bowls and spoon the rice mixture on top.

Nutrition Information (per serving):

Calories 579

Carbohydrate 38g

(Fiber 10g, Sugars 7g)

Fat 45g (Saturated Fat 24.5g)

Protein 17g

Cholesterol 11mg

Sodium 719mg

Macros: 69% Fat, 12% Protein, 19% Carbs

Net Carbs: 28g

Smoked Trout and Avocado Rice Bowls

SERVES 2 • TOTAL TIME: 15 MINUTES

⅔ cup cold cooked white rice

¼ cup chopped fresh cilantro or green onions

2 teaspoons sesame seeds, toasted

2 tablespoons coconut aminos

2 tablespoons toasted sesame oil

1 teaspoon grated fresh ginger

2 teaspoons hot sauce, or to taste

1 avocado, pitted, peeled, and chopped

2 ounces smoked trout fillets, broken into bite-size pieces

¼ cup slivered almonds, toasted

½ cup fresh pineapple chunks, chopped into ½-inch pieces

2 lime wedges

1. Divide the rice between 2 bowls. Top with the cilantro and sesame seeds.

2. In a small bowl, whisk together coconut aminos, sesame oil, ginger, and hot sauce. Spoon the sauce evenly over the rice mixture.

3. Arrange the avocado, trout, almonds, and pineapple in sections around (or on top of) the rice mixture. Serve with lime wedges.

Nutrition Information (per serving):

Calories 534

Carbohydrate 37g

(Fiber 10g, Sugars 6g)

Fat 40g (Saturated Fat 5.4g)

Protein 16g

Cholesterol 40mg

Sodium 475mg

Macros: 68% Fat, 12% Protein, 20% Carbs

Net Carbs: 27g

Taco Cauliflower Bowl

SERVES 1 • PREP: 15 MINUTES • COOK: 3 MINUTES

1 tablespoon avocado oil

2 cups freshly riced cauliflower

¾ teaspoon chili powder

¼ teaspoon ground cumin

⅛ teaspoon sea salt

⅛ teaspoon black pepper

1 lime wedge

¼ cup grape tomatoes, halved

2 tablespoons sliced radishes

½ small avocado, pitted, peeled, and sliced

2 tablespoons pumpkin seeds (pepitas)

2 tablespoons chopped Spanish (manzanilla) olives

1 tablespoon chopped fresh cilantro

1. In a medium skillet, heat the avocado oil over medium-high heat. Add the cauliflower, chili powder, cumin, salt, and pepper. Sauté 3 to 5 minutes or until the cauliflower is tender and starting to brown. Squeeze lime juice from the wedge over cauliflower and stir to combine. Transfer to a medium bowl.

2. Arrange the tomatoes, radishes, avocado slices, pumpkin seeds, and olives over the cauliflower. Top with cilantro.

Nutrition Information (per serving):

Calories 404

Carbohydrate 24g

(Fiber 11g, Sugars 6g)

Fat 34g (Saturated Fat 5g)

Protein 11g

Cholesterol 0mg

Sodium 792mg

Macros: 76% Fat, 11% Protein, 13% Carbs

Net Carbs: 14g

Turmeric-Rubbed Chicken

SERVES: 1 • **PREP: 5 MINUTES** • **COOK: 5 MINUTES**

⅛ teaspoon ground turmeric

⅛ teaspoon ground cumin

⅛ teaspoon sea salt

Pinch of cayenne pepper

Pinch of ground coriander

Pinch of ground ginger

1 boneless, skinless chicken breast (4 ounces)

1 tablespoon coconut oil

Lime wedge

1. In a small bowl, combine the turmeric, cumin, salt, cayenne pepper, coriander, and ginger. Rub over the chicken.

2. In a small skillet, heat the coconut oil over medium-high heat. Add the chicken to the skillet; cook 5 to 6 minutes per side or until no longer pink in the center. Serve with lime wedge.

Nutrition Information (per serving):

Calories 256

Carbohydrate 0g

(Fiber 0g, Sugars 0g)

Fat 17g (Saturated Fat 12.5g)

Protein 26g

Cholesterol 83mg

Sodium 342mg

Macros: 60% Fat, 40% Protein, 0% Carbs

Net Carbs: 0g

Spinach + Ricotta Portobello Caps

SERVES 2 • PREP: 15 MINUTES • COOK: 25 MINUTES

4 large portobello caps (about 12 ounces total), wiped clean with a damp cloth

Avocado oil cooking spray

½ cup vegan ricotta cheese

2 teaspoons dried oregano

⅛ teaspoon crushed red pepper flakes

¼ teaspoon kosher salt

1½ tablespoons olive oil, divided

4 ounces fresh baby spinach

⅓ cup sliced almonds

½ cup organic tomato sauce

1. Preheat oven to 425°F. Line a baking sheet with foil.

2. Coat both sides of the mushroom caps with cooking spray and place, stem side down, on the prepared baking sheet. Bake 10 minutes, turn over, and bake 5 minutes or until tender.

3. Meanwhile, in a small bowl, combine the ricotta, oregano, pepper flakes, and salt.

4. Heat a medium skillet over medium heat. Add 1 tablespoon of the oil to the skillet, and tilt to lightly coat the bottom. Add the spinach and almonds and cook 1 to 2 minutes, stirring constantly, just until spinach is wilted. Remove from heat.

5. Spoon half of the tomato sauce on top of the mushroom caps, top with equal amounts of the spinach mixture, and spoon ricotta on top of the spinach. Top with the remaining tomato sauce over all and drizzle with remaining ½ tablespoon of oil. Bake 10 minutes or until heated through.

Nutrition Information (per serving):

Calories 396

Carbohydrate 22g

(Fiber 9g, Sugars 11g)

Fat 32g (Saturated Fat 3.2g)

Protein 14g

Cholesterol 1mg

Sodium 807mg

Macros: 72% Fat, 15% Protein, 13% Carbs

Net Carbs: 13g

Lemon Chicken

SERVES 1 • PREP: 5 MINUTES • COOK: 7 MINUTES

1 tablespoon ghee, divided

1 boneless, skinless chicken breast (4 ounces)

Sea salt and black pepper

1 small garlic clove, minced

1 tablespoon fresh lemon juice

1. In a small skillet, heat ½ tablespoon of the ghee over medium-high heat. Season the chicken with a pinch each of salt and pepper. Cook the chicken 5 to 6 minutes per side or until done. Remove from the pan and keep warm.

2. Add the garlic to the pan and cook 1 minute. Add the lemon juice and remaining ½ tablespoon ghee to the pan. Cook 1 to 2 minutes, scraping the bottom of the pan to loosen the browned bits. Pour the sauce over the chicken.

Nutrition Information (per serving):

Calories 270

Carbohydrate 2g

(Fiber 0g, Sugars 0g)

Fat 20g (Saturated Fat 12g)

Protein 20g

Cholesterol 196mg

Sodium 270mg

Macros: 68% Fat, 29% Protein, 3% Carbs

Net Carbs: 0g

VQ

Skewered Tuna with Avocado Salad Salsa

SERVES 2 • PREP: 10 MINUTES • COOK: 4 MINUTES

Skewers

- Avocado oil cooking spray
- 8-ounce tuna fillet (about ¾-inch thick), rinsed and patted dry, cut into 1-inch cubes
- 8 grape tomatoes
- 1 tablespoon avocado oil
- ⅛ teaspoon kosher salt
- Black pepper to taste

Avocado Salad Salsa

- ⅔ cup chopped cucumber
- ¼ cup finely chopped red onion
- ¼ cup chopped fresh cilantro
- 2 tablespoons extra-virgin olive oil
- 2 tablespoons fresh lemon juice
- ⅛ teaspoon crushed red pepper flakes
- ¼ teaspoon kosher salt
- 1 avocado, pitted, peeled, and chopped
- 2 lemon wedges

1. To make the skewers: Preheat grill or grill pan coated with avocado oil cooking spray to medium-high heat.

2. Alternately thread two 10- to 12-inch skewers with tuna and tomatoes. Brush tuna and tomatoes with the avocado oil and sprinkle evenly with the salt and black pepper. Cook 2 minutes, turn, and cook 1½ to 2 minutes or to desired doneness. (Do not overcook or it will be tough and dry. Tuna should be very rare for peak tenderness and flavor.)

3. To make the salad: In a medium bowl, combine the cucumber, onion, cilantro, olive oil, lemon juice, pepper flakes, and the salt. Gently stir in the avocado.

4. Divide the avocado mixture between 2 plates, place the skewers alongside, and squeeze the lemon over the tuna and tomatoes.

Nutrition Information (per serving):

Calories 440
Carbohydrate 13g
(Fiber 6g, Sugars 4g)
Fat 32g (Saturated Fat 4.5g)
Protein 30g

Cholesterol 44mg
Sodium 423mg
Macros: 66% Fat, 27% Protein, 7% Carbs
Net Carbs: 7g

Poached Eggs with Tarragon Sauce and Asparagus

SERVES 2 • **PREP: 8 MINUTES** • **COOK: 8 MINUTES**

Sauce

- ⅓ cup unsweetened plain vegan yogurt
- 2 tablespoons avocado oil mayonnaise
- 1 to 1½ teaspoons no-sugar-added whole-grain mustard, to taste
- 1 teaspoon chopped fresh tarragon or ¼ teaspoon dried
- ¼ teaspoon kosher salt

Eggs and Vegetables

- 4 large eggs
- 2 teaspoons white vinegar
- 8 ounces asparagus spears, trimmed
- 1 cup frozen green peas
- Kosher salt and black pepper

1. To make the sauce: In a small bowl, whisk together the yogurt, mayonnaise, 1 to 2 tablespoons water (depending on desired consistency), mustard, tarragon, and salt; set aside.

2. Break each egg into a separate custard cup or ramekin. Fill a large skillet two-thirds full with water. Add the vinegar and bring to a simmer. Pour each egg gently into the skillet. Turn off the heat, cover, and let stand 5 minutes. Do *not* remove lid during this time.

3. Meanwhile, place the asparagus in a microwave-safe dish, such as a glass pie dish. Add ½ cup water, cover, and microwave 2 minutes. Add the peas, and continue to cook, uncovered, in 1-minute increments, until the asparagus is tender crisp.

4. Remove the asparagus with tongs and divide them between 2 plates. Spoon equal amounts of the sauce across the center of the asparagus. Drain the peas well and spoon over the asparagus. Cover to keep warm.

5. Carefully remove the eggs with a slotted spoon. Top each plate with 2 eggs. Sprinkle with salt and pepper to taste.

Nutrition Information (per serving):

Calories 343
Carbohydrate 17g
(Fiber 6g, Sugars 6g)
Fat 25g (Saturated Fat 5g)
Protein 20g

Cholesterol 375mg
Sodium 495mg
Macros: 65% Fat, 23% Protein, 12% Carbs
Net Carbs: 11g

Homestyle Meatloaf and Roasted Beans

SERVES 2 • PREP: 10 MINUTES • COOK: 50 MINUTES

3 tablespoons avocado oil, divided

½ cup organic tomato sauce

2 teaspoons coconut aminos

½ teaspoon hot sauce

Kosher salt and black pepper

8 ounces 93% lean grass-fed ground sirloin

⅓ cup chopped onion

⅓ cup chopped poblano chile pepper

2 egg yolks

¼ cup almond flour

½ teaspoon dried oregano

2 teaspoons balsamic vinegar

2 drops liquid stevia

8 ounces whole green beans, stemmed

1. Preheat oven to 350°F. Line a baking sheet with foil and coat it with 1 tablespoon of the oil.

2. In a small bowl, whisk together the tomato sauce, 1 tablespoon of the oil, the coconut aminos, hot sauce, ⅛ teaspoon salt, and black pepper to taste.

3. In a medium bowl, combine the beef, onion, poblano pepper, egg yolks, flour, oregano, and half of the tomato sauce mixture. Mix until just blended. Be careful not to overmix.

4. Place the beef mixture on the prepared baking sheet and shape into an oval loaf, about 4 inches by 3 inches. Bake for 25 minutes.

5. Stir the vinegar and stevia into the remaining tomato sauce mixture and spoon evenly over the top and sides of the meatloaf. Toss the green beans with the remaining 1 tablespoon oil and ⅛ teaspoon salt. Arrange the beans in a single layer around the meatloaf. Bake for 25 minutes or until the meatloaf is no longer pink in the center.

6. Let stand 5 minutes before slicing. Divide the meatloaf slices and beans between 2 plates. Season with salt and pepper to taste.

Nutrition Information (per serving):

Calories 490	Cholesterol 256mg
Carbohydrate 20	Sodium 834mg
(Fiber 6g, Sugars 9g)	**Macros:** 62% Fat, 27% Protein,
Fat 34g (Saturated Fat 7.1g)	11% Carbs
Protein 33g	**Net Carbs:** 14g

Grilled Salmon with Fresh Orange + Chia Seed Salsa

SERVES 2 • PREP: 10 MINUTES • COOK: 6 MINUTES

¼ to ½ teaspoon grated orange zest

½ cup chopped fresh orange sections

¼ cup finely chopped red bell pepper

¼ cup finely chopped red onion

2 tablespoons unsweetened dried coconut flakes

¼ teaspoon chia seeds

⅛ teaspoon crushed red pepper flakes

1 teaspoon balsamic vinegar

1 or 2 drops liquid stevia (optional)

2 tablespoons coconut aminos

2 tablespoons toasted sesame oil

8-ounce fresh skinless salmon fillet, rinsed and patted dry

⅛ teaspoon kosher salt

Black pepper

1. Preheat grill to medium-high heat.

2. In a medium bowl, combine the orange zest, oranges, bell pepper, onion, coconut flakes, chia seeds, pepper flakes, vinegar, and stevia, if using.

3. In a small bowl, whisk together the coconut aminos and sesame oil. Reserve 2 tablespoons and brush the remaining mixture on both sides of the salmon; sprinkle with the salt and black pepper to taste.

4. Place the salmon on the grill; cook 3 minutes and then turn and cook an additional 3 minutes or until the salmon flakes with a fork.

5. Cut the salmon in half and divide between 2 plates. Spoon the reserved coconut aminos mixture over the salmon and serve the salsa on top or alongside.

Nutrition Information (per serving):

Calories 430

Carbohydrate 13g

(Fiber 2g, Sugars 6g)

Fat 32g (Saturated Fat 7.9g)

Protein 24g

Cholesterol 62mg

Sodium 649mg

Macros: 67% Fat, 23% Protein, 10% Carbs

Net Carbs: 11g

Veggie Frittata with Lemon-Splashed Spring Greens

SERVES 2 • PREP: 8 MINUTES • COOK: 15 MINUTES

5 large eggs

¼ cup unsweetened almond milk

½ teaspoon dried oregano

Kosher salt and black pepper

2 tablespoons olive oil, divided

1 cup thinly sliced zucchini

⅓ cup chopped red bell pepper

2 garlic cloves, minced

½ (14-ounce) can quartered artichoke hearts, drained and coarsely chopped

1 medium green onion, finely chopped

2 ounces vegan feta cheese, crumbled

2 cups spring greens

2 teaspoons fresh lemon juice

1. In a medium bowl, whisk together the eggs, almond milk, oregano, ⅛ teaspoon salt, and black pepper to taste. Set aside.

2. In a medium nonstick skillet, heat 1 tablespoon of oil over medium-high heat. Cook zucchini and bell pepper for 3 to 4 minutes or until lightly browned, stirring occasionally. Add garlic and cook 15 seconds, stirring constantly.

3. Reduce heat to medium, stir in the artichokes, and spread evenly over the bottom of the skillet. Sprinkle with the green onion. Reduce heat to medium-low. Carefully pour egg mixture over all and cover and cook 10 minutes or just until set. Remove from heat, sprinkle with cheese, cover, and let stand for 5 minutes.

4. Toss the spring greens with remaining 1 tablespoon of oil, lemon juice, and salt and pepper to taste.

5. Cut the frittata into wedges, divide between 2 plates, and top with the spring greens.

Nutrition Information (per serving):

Calories 454

Carbohydrate 19g

(Fiber 4g, Sugars 3g)

Fat 35g (Saturated Fat 12.9g)

Protein 21g

Cholesterol 465mg

Sodium 976mg

Macros: 69% Fat, 18% Protein, 13% Carbs

Net Carbs: 15g

Spicy Sauced Beef Tips

SERVES 2 • **PREP: 5 MINUTES** • **COOK: 12 MINUTES**

3 tablespoons olive oil, divided

8 ounces grass-fed boneless beef, such as sirloin or rib-eye, cut into 1-inch cubes and patted dry

Black pepper

¾ cup thinly sliced onion

¾ cup chopped tomato

¼ cup red wine

12 pitted kalamata olives

½ cup organic medium salsa, such as Newman's Own

1 tablespoon chopped fresh oregano

Kosher salt

1. In a large skillet, heat 1 tablespoon of oil over medium-high until hot. Sprinkle beef lightly with black pepper on both sides to taste. Add beef to the skillet and cook for 4 to 5 minutes, or until beginning to brown, stirring occasionally. Set aside on a plate.

2. Add the onion to the skillet and cook, stirring occasionally, for 3 to 4 minutes or until golden. Add the tomatoes, wine, and olives; cook 2 to 3 minutes, stirring occasionally, or until liquid evaporates. Add the salsa and oregano. Bring to a boil and then reduce heat to medium. Add the meat to the skillet along with any accumulated juices and remaining 2 tablespoons of oil; cook and stir for 1 minute to heat through. Season with salt and pepper to taste.

3. Divide between 2 shallow bowls.

Nutrition Information (per serving):

Calories 437

Carbohydrate 15g

(Fiber 4g, Sugars 6g)

Fat 32g (Saturated Fat 5.4g)

Protein 27g

Cholesterol 68mg

Sodium 647mg

Macros: 66% Fat, 24% Protein, 10% Carbs

Net Carbs: 11g

Herbed-Ghee Marinated Chicken with Broccoli

**SERVES 2 • PREP: 6 MINUTES (PLUS 2 HOURS MARINATING TIME) •
COOK: 10 MINUTES**

2 boneless, skinless
chicken breasts
(4 ounces each)

¼ cup ghee

1 teaspoon grated lemon
zest

1½ tablespoons fresh
lemon juice

1 green onion, minced

1 garlic clove, minced

1 teaspoon dried basil

½ teaspoon dried dill

½ teaspoon kosher salt

3 cups broccoli florets

2 lemon wedges

1. Place the chicken breasts in a single layer between 2 sheets of plastic wrap. Using a meat pounder or bottom of a can, flatten the chicken breasts to a ¼-inch thickness.

2. In a small bowl, combine the ghee, lemon zest, lemon juice, green onion, garlic, basil, dill, and salt. Stir until well blended. Coat both sides of the chicken with the ghee mixture. Place in a shallow pan or rimmed plate. Cover and refrigerate overnight or at least 2 hours.

3. Place ¾ cup water and the broccoli in a medium skillet. Bring to a boil, reduce heat, cover, and simmer for 3 to 4 minutes or until the broccoli is tender crisp. Drain and divide between 2 plates. Cover to keep warm.

4. Dry the skillet with a paper towel and return to medium-high heat. Add the chicken and ghee mixture and cook for 3 minutes on each side or until the chicken is no longer pink in the center. Place on two plates.

5. Add ¼ cup water to the pan drippings in the skillet and boil for 1 minute or until thickened slightly. Pour the sauce over the chicken and serve with lemon wedges.

Nutrition Information (per serving):

Calories 417

Carbohydrate 8g

(Fiber 3g, Sugars 1g)

Fat 31g (Saturated Fat 17.5g)

Protein 29g

Cholesterol 127mg

Sodium 561mg

Macros: 68% Fat, 28% Protein,
4% Carbs

Net Carbs: 5g

Stuffed Squash with Cream Cheese

SERVES 2 • PREP: 12 MINUTES • COOK: 25 MINUTES

1 tablespoon plus
    1 teaspoon olive oil,
    divided

2 crookneck squash
    (about 14 ounces total),
    halved lengthwise

1 green onion, chopped

¼ cup finely chopped
    poblano chile pepper

2 tablespoons chopped
    fresh parsley

1 garlic clove, minced

⅓ cup vegan cream
    cheese

½ teaspoon kosher salt,
    divided

Paprika to taste

3 cups shredded mustard
    greens or baby kale mix

2 teaspoons hot sauce

Black pepper

2 tablespoons finely
    chopped walnuts

1. Preheat the oven to 450°F. Line a baking sheet with foil and coat with 1 teaspoon of the olive oil.

2. Using a spoon, scoop the pulp out of the squash halves.

3. Coarsely chop the pulp and place in a medium bowl with the green onion, poblano pepper, parsley, garlic, cream cheese, and ¼ teaspoon of salt. Stir until well blended. Spoon the mixture into the squash, pressing down lightly to adhere, and sprinkle lightly with paprika. Place on the prepared baking sheet. Drizzle with 1 tablespoon olive oil and bake 25 to 30 minutes or until squash is just tender.

4. In a medium bowl, combine the mustard greens, remaining 1 tablespoon of olive oil, and the hot sauce. Toss until well coated and sprinkle with the remaining ¼ teaspoon salt and black pepper to taste.

5. Divide greens between 2 plates, sprinkle with walnuts, and top with the squash halves.

Nutrition Information (per serving):

Calories 325

Carbohydrate 18g

(Fiber 6g, Sugars 7g)

Fat 27g (Saturated Fat 4.5g)

Protein 9g

Cholesterol 0mg

Sodium 373mg

Macros: 74% Fat, 11% Protein, 15% Carbs

Net Carbs: 12g

Sheet Pan Pecan-Crusted Cod and Carrots

SERVES 2 • PREP: 10 MINUTES • COOK: 30 MINUTES

3 medium carrots, quartered lengthwise and cut into 2-inch pieces

⅓ cup chopped onion

2 tablespoons coconut oil, divided

¼ teaspoon kosher salt, divided

Black pepper to taste

1 tablespoon coconut aminos

¼ teaspoon cider vinegar

½ teaspoon hot sauce

6 drops liquid stevia

2 cod fillets (4 ounces each), rinsed and patted dry

¼ cup finely chopped pecans

1. Preheat oven to 400° F. Line a baking sheet with foil.

2. Place the carrots and onion on the prepared baking sheet. Toss with 1 tablespoon of the coconut oil and arrange in a single layer. Sprinkle with ⅛ teaspoon of salt and black pepper. Bake for 20 minutes.

3. Meanwhile, in a small bowl, whisk together the coconut aminos, vinegar, hot sauce, stevia, and remaining 1 tablespoon of oil. Set aside.

4. Move the carrots to one side of the baking sheet. Arrange the fish fillets on the other side of the baking sheet. Spoon the coconut aminos mixture evenly over the top of the fillets and carefully mound the pecans on top. Bake for 10 to 12 minutes or until fish flakes easily with a fork. Serve with the carrots, scraping any remaining nuts and sauce from the baking sheet onto the fish.

Nutrition Information (per serving):

Calories 360

Carbohydrate 17g

(Fiber 5g, Sugars 7g)

Fat 25g (Saturated Fat 12.8g)

Protein 23g

Cholesterol 49mg

Sodium 612mg

Macros: 61% Fat, 25% Protein, 14% Carbs

Net Carbs: 12g

Walnut Portobellos in Sage Butter

SERVES 2 • PREP: 8 MINUTES • COOK: 15 MINUTES

1 bunch broccolini (about 8 ounces), ends trimmed, and cut in half lengthwise

3 tablespoons ghee, divided

12 ounces portobello mushroom caps, cut into ¼-inch-thick slices

¼ cup chopped walnuts

2 garlic cloves, peeled and crushed

10 fresh sage leaves

Kosher salt and black pepper

1 teaspoon balsamic vinegar

1. In a large skillet, bring 2 to 3 inches of water to boil over high heat. Add the broccolini and cook 2 minutes or until bright green and tender crisp. Drain well in a colander and set aside.

2. Dry the skillet with a paper towel. Reduce heat to medium-high and add 1 tablespoon of ghee. When melted, add half of the mushrooms and cook, stirring occasionally, 5 to 7 minutes or until tender. Set aside on a plate. Repeat with 1 tablespoon of ghee and the remaining mushrooms and set aside on the same plate.

3. Heat the remaining 1 tablespoon of ghee in the skillet. Reduce heat to medium-low heat. When melted, add walnuts and garlic and cook, stirring frequently, 3 to 4 minutes or until beginning to lightly brown. Add the sage leaves and cook for 1 minute or until the sage begins to darken and crisp. Add the mushrooms, ½ teaspoon salt, black pepper to taste, and the vinegar. Stir and cook 1 minute or until heated through. Remove from heat.

4. Divide the broccolini between 2 plates. Sprinkle lightly with salt and pepper to taste. Top with equal amounts of the mushroom mixture.

Nutrition Information (per serving):

Calories 365
Carbohydrate 17g
(Fiber 6g, Sugars 7g)
Fat 32g (Saturated Fat 13.7g)
Protein 9g

Cholesterol 34mg
Sodium 534mg
Macros: 78% Fat, 10% Protein, 12% Carbs
Net Carbs: 11g

Spinach-Artichoke Turmeric Rice

SERVES 2 • **PREP: 5 MINUTES** • **COOK: 25 MINUTES**

¼ cup olive oil, divided

½ cup pumpkin seeds (pepitas)

½ cup chopped green bell pepper

½ (14-ounce) can quartered artichoke hearts, drained

2 garlic cloves, minced

¼ cup uncooked white rice or Arborio rice

½ teaspoon paprika

¼ teaspoon ground turmeric

¼ teaspoon kosher salt

2 cups chopped fresh spinach

¼ cup chopped tomatoes

Black pepper to taste

8 small pitted ripe olives, coarsely chopped

1. Heat 2 tablespoons of oil in a medium skillet over medium-high heat. Add pumpkin seeds and cook for 1 to 2 minutes, or until beginning to lightly brown. Remove with a slotted spoon and set aside on a plate. To the skillet, add the bell peppers, artichokes, and garlic and cook for 5 minutes. Add ¾ cup water, rice, paprika, turmeric, and salt. Bring to a boil, reduce heat, cover, and simmer for 18 minutes or until rice is tender.

2. Remove from the heat and stir in the spinach, tomatoes, and remaining 2 tablespoons of oil. Sprinkle with black pepper and olives. Let stand 10 minutes to absorb the flavors.

Nutrition Information (per serving):

Calories 567

Carbohydrate 35g

(Fiber 6g, Sugars 2g)

Fat 44g (Saturated Fat 6.6g)

Protein 14g

Cholesterol 0mg

Sodium 730mg

Macros: 70% Fat, 10% Protein, 20% Carbs

Net Carbs: 29g

Sesame Thai Toss with Citrus–Nut Butter Sauce

SERVES 2 • PREP: 10 MINUTES • COOK: 8 MINUTES

Sauce

- 2 tablespoons almond butter
- 2 tablespoons coconut aminos
- 2 tablespoons fresh lime juice
- 2 to 4 drops liquid stevia, or to taste
- ⅛ teaspoon crushed red pepper flakes

Base

- ½ cup peanuts or slivered almonds
- 1 tablespoon sesame seeds
- 1 tablespoon toasted sesame oil
- 2 cups small cauliflower florets, about ½-inch diameter
- 2 cups small broccoli florets
- 1½ cups matchstick carrots
- ½ red bell pepper, thinly sliced
- ⅓ cup frozen green peas, thawed
- ¼ teaspoon kosher salt
- 1 medium green onion, chopped
- ¼ cup chopped fresh cilantro
- 2 lime wedges

1. To make the sauce: Place the almond butter and coconut aminos in a small microwave-safe bowl and microwave for 20 to 25 seconds on high. Whisk until well blended and stir in the lime juice, 2 to 3 tablespoons of water (depending on desired consistency), the stevia, and pepper flakes. Set aside.

2. To make the base: Heat a large skillet over medium-high heat. Add the nuts and cook for 2 minutes, stirring frequently. Add the sesame seeds and cook for 1 minute, stirring constantly. Set aside on a plate. Add the sesame oil and tilt skillet to lightly coat the bottom. Stir in the cauliflower, broccoli, carrots, bell pepper, peas, and salt; cook for 3 minutes or until carrots are slightly limp, stirring frequently. Remove from heat.

3. Spoon the sauce evenly over the cauliflower mixture, and then sprinkle with nuts, sesame seeds, green onion, and cilantro. Serve as is or toss gently. Serve with lime wedges alongside.

Nutrition Information (per serving):

Calories 520
Carbohydrate 39g
(Fiber 14g, Sugars 12g)
Fat 38g (Saturated Fat 5.5g)
Protein 20g

Cholesterol 0mg
Sodium 353mg
Macros: 65% Fat, 15% Protein, 20% Carbs
Net Carbs: 25g

Catfish with Rustic Creole Sauce

SERVES 2 • **PREP: 5 MINUTES** • **COOK: 15 MINUTES**

¼ cup ghee, divided

1 cup finely chopped green bell pepper

1 medium celery stalk, thinly sliced

½ cup finely chopped onion

½ teaspoon dried thyme

⅛ teaspoon cayenne pepper

1 small tomato, chopped

2 tablespoons chopped fresh parsley

2 teaspoons fresh lemon juice

½ teaspoon kosher salt, divided

8 ounces catfish fillet

Black pepper

⅔ cup cooked white rice

2 lemon wedges

1. Heat a large skillet over medium-high heat and add 2 tablespoons of the ghee. When melted, add bell peppers, celery, onions, thyme, and cayenne; cook for 5 to 6 minutes or until beginning to lightly brown, stirring occasionally. Add the tomato and cook for 2 minutes or until slightly softened. Stir in the parsley, lemon juice, and ¼ teaspoon salt. Set aside in a bowl and cover to keep warm.

2. In the same skillet, heat the remaining 2 tablespoons of ghee over medium-high heat. When melted, tilt skillet to lightly coat the bottom. Sprinkle both sides of the fish with the remaining ¼ teaspoon salt and black pepper to taste. Add to the pan and cook 3 minutes on one side; then turn and cook 2 minutes or until opaque in the center. Remove from the heat.

3. Divide the rice between 2 plates, spoon the sauce over the rice, and top with fish. Serve with lemon wedges.

Nutrition Information (per serving):

Calories 489
Carbohydrate 26g
(Fiber 4g, Sugars 5.5g)
Fat 35g (Saturated Fat 18.4g)
Protein 21g

Cholesterol 107mg
Sodium 621mg
Macros: 65% Fat, 17% Protein, 18% Carbs
Net Carbs: 22g

Sweet Potato Patties with Spicy Yogurt

SERVES 2 • PREP: 10 MINUTES • COOK: 10 MINUTES

Topping

- ¼ cup unsweetened plain vegan yogurt
- ½ teaspoon hot sauce
- ⅛ teaspoon kosher salt
- ¼ cup pumpkin seeds
- ¼ cup hemp seeds

Patties

- 2 medium sweet potatoes
- ½ of a small onion
- 1 large egg, lightly beaten
- 1 tablespoon avocado oil mayonnaise
- 1 garlic clove, minced
- 1 teaspoon ground cumin
- ½ teaspoon smoked paprika
- ¼ teaspoon kosher salt
- 2 tablespoons coconut oil
- 1 tablespoon chopped fresh parsley

1. In a small bowl, combine the yogurt, hot sauce, and salt. Set aside.

2. Heat a large skillet over medium-high heat until hot. Add the pumpkin seeds and hemp seeds and cook for 2 to 3 minutes or until beginning to lightly brown, stirring frequently. Set aside on a plate.

3. Shred the sweet potatoes and onion in a food processor using the large shredder side of the blade. In a medium bowl, combine the potatoes and onion with the egg, mayonnaise, garlic, cumin, paprika, and salt.

4. Heat the coconut oil in a large skillet over medium heat. Spoon ¼ cup of the potato mixture into the skillet and flatten into a ½-inch-thick patty (about 3 inches in diameter). Repeat with remaining mixture to make 3 more patties.

5. Cook for 3 to 4 minutes on each side or until golden brown, gently turning using a flat spatula.

6. Divide between 2 plates, sprinkle parsley and seeds over the patties, and top with the yogurt mixture.

Nutrition Information (per serving):

Calories 564
Carbohydrate 31g
(Fiber 6g, Sugars 7g)
Fat 43g (Saturated Fat 17g)
Protein 20g

Cholesterol 101mg
Sodium 530mg
Macros: 68% Fat, 14% Protein, 18% Carbs
Net Carbs: 25g

Veggie Skillet with Mozzarella

SERVES 2 • PREP: 7 MINUTES • COOK: 10 MINUTES

3 tablespoons avocado oil

½ cup chopped onion

½ cup chopped green bell pepper

4 ounces sliced mushrooms

1 medium crookneck squash, chopped

2 garlic cloves, minced

½ (15-ounce) can organic kidney beans, rinsed and drained

2 teaspoons spirulina powder

1½ teaspoons chili powder

1 teaspoon ground cumin

⅛ teaspoon crushed red pepper flakes

¼ teaspoon kosher salt

Black pepper to taste

⅓ cup chopped fresh cilantro

4 ounces vegan mozzarella cheese, shredded

1. Heat oil in a medium skillet over medium-high heat. Tilt skillet to lightly coat the bottom, and then cook the onions and peppers for 4 minutes, stirring occasionally, or until beginning to lightly brown. Add the mushrooms, squash, and garlic to the skillet, and cook, stirring occasionally, for 4 to 5 minutes or until the vegetables are just tender. Add the kidney beans, spirulina, chili powder, cumin, pepper flakes, salt, black pepper, and cilantro. Cook and stir for 2 to 3 minutes to heat through.

2. Divide between 2 plates and sprinkle with the cheese.

Nutrition Information (per serving):

Calories 459

Carbohydrate 29g

(Fiber 6g, Sugars 8g)

Fat 36g (Saturated Fat 12.7g)

Protein 10g

Cholesterol 0mg

Sodium 783mg

Macros: 71% Fat, 9% Protein, 20% Carbs

Net Carbs: 23g

Garlic Asparagus + Lentil Pasta

SERVES 2 • **PREP: 5 MINUTES** • **COOK: 15 MINUTES**

¾ cup uncooked lentil pasta

1 cup asparagus spears, cut into 2-inch pieces

¼ cup ghee, divided

8 ounces mixed exotic fresh mushrooms, coarsely chopped

3 to 4 garlic cloves, minced

1 tablespoon chopped fresh oregano

½ teaspoon kosher salt

Black pepper to taste

1. Cook the pasta according to package directions. Add the asparagus 3 minutes before the end of cooking time.

2. Meanwhile, heat a large skillet over medium-high heat. Once hot, add 2 tablespoons of the ghee. Tilt skillet to lightly coat the bottom. Add the mushrooms and cook for 5 to 7 minutes, stirring occasionally, or until tender. Stir in the garlic and oregano. Cook for 15 seconds, stirring constantly.

3. Drain the pasta mixture and add to the mushrooms, with the remaining ghee and the salt. Toss until well blended.

4. Divide between 2 plates. Sprinkle with black pepper.

Nutrition Information (per serving):

Calories 382

Carbohydrate 25g

(Fiber 6g, Sugars 4g)

Fat 29g (Saturated Fat 16.9g)

Protein 10g

Cholesterol 45mg

Sodium 492mg

Macros: 69% Fat, 11% Protein, 20% Carbs

Net Carbs: 19g

Kale, Brussels Sprout, and Blueberry Salad

SERVES 2 • TOTAL TIME: 15 MINUTES

Salad

1½ cups chopped kale

1½ cups shredded Brussels
    sprouts

⅓ cup sunflower seeds,
    toasted

1 jalapeño pepper,
    seeded (if desired) and
    finely chopped

Dressing

¼ cup extra-virgin olive oil

1 teaspoon grated lemon
    zest

1 tablespoon fresh lemon
    juice

1 tablespoon no-sugar-
    added whole-grain
    mustard

1 garlic clove, minced

¼ teaspoon kosher salt

4 to 6 drops liquid stevia,
    or to taste

½ cup blueberries

1. To make the salad: In a large bowl, combine the kale, Brussels sprouts, sunflower seeds, and jalapeño.

2. To make the dressing: In a small bowl, whisk together the olive oil, lemon zest, lemon juice, mustard, garlic, salt, and liquid stevia until well blended.

3. Pour the dressing over the kale mixture and toss until well coated. Add the blueberries and toss gently. Divide between 2 plates.

Nutrition Information (per serving):

Calories 447

Carbohydrate 22g

(Fiber 7g, Sugars 6g)

Fat 39g (Saturated Fat 4.9g)

Protein 8g

Cholesterol 0mg

Sodium 377mg

Macros: 79% Fat, 7% Protein, 14% Carbs

Net Carbs: 15g

Pepperoncini Tomato Salad

SERVES 2 • TOTAL TIME: 10 MINUTES

1 cup grape tomatoes, halved

½ cup chopped cucumber

10 pitted large ripe olives, halved

3 pepperoncini peppers, sliced

1 ounce vegan mozzarella cheese, chopped

2 to 3 teaspoons chopped fresh oregano

1 tablespoon extra-virgin olive oil

2 teaspoons apple cider vinegar

Kosher salt and black pepper

2 cups baby kale mixed greens

In a medium bowl, combine the grape tomatoes, cucumber, olives, peppers, mozzarella, oregano, olive oil, and cider vinegar. Add salt and pepper to taste. Divide the mixed greens between 2 plates and top with the tomato mixture.

Nutrition Information (per serving):

Calories 152

Carbohydrate 9g

(Fiber 3g, Sugars 2g)

Fat 13g (Saturated Fat 4g)

Protein 3g

Cholesterol 0mg

Sodium 427mg

Macros: 78% Fat, 7% Protein, 15% Carbs

Net Carbs: 6g

Jicama and Fresh Mint Salad

SERVES 2 • **PREP: 12 MINUTES** • **STAND: 15 MINUTES**

8 ounces jicama, peeled, thinly sliced, and cut into matchstick-size pieces (about 1½ cups total)

⅓ cup diced radishes

¼ cup chopped fresh mint

1 teaspoon grated lemon zest

3 tablespoons fresh lemon juice

1 teaspoon grated fresh ginger

9 to 12 drops liquid stevia, or to taste

1 avocado, pitted, peeled, and sliced

1. In a medium bowl, stir together the jicama, radishes, mint, lemon zest, lemon juice, ginger, and liquid stevia. Let stand 15 minutes to absorb flavors.

2. To serve, divide the jicama mixture between 2 salad plates. Arrange avocado slices alongside.

Nutrition Information (per serving):

Calories 328

Carbohydrate 30g

(Fiber 20g, Sugars 4g)

Fat 30g (Saturated Fat 4.3g)

Protein 5g

Cholesterol 0mg

Sodium 29mg

Macros: 81% Fat, 7% Protein, 12% Carbs

Net Carbs: 10g

Arugula Salad

SERVES 1 • **TOTAL TIME: 5 MINUTES**

1½ cups baby arugula

2 tablespoons pumpkin seeds (pepitas), toasted

1 tablespoon extra-virgin olive oil

1 tablespoon fresh lemon juice

1 teaspoon nutritional yeast

Sea salt and black pepper

1. In a medium bowl, combine the arugula and pumpkin seeds.

2. In a small bowl, whisk together the olive oil, lemon juice, nutritional yeast, and a pinch each of salt and pepper. Drizzle over the arugula mixture.

Nutrition Information (per serving):

Calories 231
Carbohydrate 5g
(Fiber 2g, Sugars 2g)
Fat 22g (Saturated Fat 3.5g)
Protein 6g

Cholesterol 0mg
Sodium 169mg
Macros: 85% Fat, 10% Protein, 5% Carbs
Net Carbs: 3g

Pickled Carrot Sticks

SERVES 1 • **TOTAL TIME: 2 HOURS 15 MINUTES**

3 carrots, peeled and cut into sticks

1½ tablespoons extra-virgin olive oil

1½ tablespoons apple cider vinegar

¼ teaspoon kosher salt

Dried drill or thyme (optional)

1. In a small jar with a lid or a small bowl, combine carrots, olive oil, vinegar, salt, and a pinch of dried herb, if desired.

2. Cover and refrigerate at least 2 hours or until ready to serve, stirring or shaking occasionally.

Nutrition Information (per serving):

Calories 249
Carbohydrate 18g
(Fiber 5g, Sugars 9g)
Fat 21g (Saturated Fat 3g)
Protein 2g

Cholesterol 0mg
Sodium 606mg
Macros: 77% Fat, 3% Protein, 20% Carbs
Net Carbs: 13g

Greens and Berry Salad with Chia Seed Dressing

SERVES 2 • TOTAL TIME: 10 MINUTES

Dressing

- 1½ tablespoons avocado oil
- 1 tablespoon white balsamic vinegar
- 1 teaspoon chia seeds
- ½ teaspoon grated fresh ginger
- 4 to 6 drops liquid stevia, or to taste
- ⅛ teaspoon kosher salt

Salad

- 2 cups baby kale mix
- 2 tablespoons finely chopped red onion
- ⅔ cup strawberries, quartered

1. In a small bowl, combine the avocado oil, white balsamic vinegar, chia seeds, ginger, liquid stevia, and salt. Let stand for 5 minutes and whisk until well blended.

2. In a salad bowl, combine the baby kale mix, onions, and dressing, and toss until it is well coated. Add the strawberries and toss gently. Divide the salad between 2 plates and serve.

Nutrition Information (per serving):

Calories 127
Carbohydrate 8g
(Fiber 3g, Sugars 4g)
Fat 11g (Saturated Fat 1.4g)
Protein 2g

Cholesterol 0mg
Sodium 140mg
Macros: 80% Fat, 5% Protein, 15% Carbs
Net Carbs: 5g

Broccoli-Mushroom Roast with Sesame Seeds

SERVES 2 • **PREP: 10 MINUTES** • **ROAST: 28 MINUTES**

- 2 cups broccoli florets
- 4 ounces baby portobello (cremini) mushrooms
- ½ cup coarsely chopped onion
- 2 tablespoons avocado oil
- ⅛ teaspoon crushed red pepper flakes
- ⅛ teaspoon kosher salt
- 1 tablespoon sesame seeds
- 1 tablespoon fresh lime juice
- 1 tablespoon coconut aminos
- 1 or 2 drops liquid stevia, or to taste

1. Preheat the oven to 425°F. Line a baking sheet with foil.

2. Place the broccoli, mushrooms, and onions on the prepared baking sheet. Toss with the oil, pepper flakes, and salt and roast for 25 minutes. Stir the mixture, sprinkle with the sesame seeds, and roast for 3 to 5 minutes more or until the broccoli is tender.

3. In a small bowl, combine the lime juice, coconut aminos, and stevia.

4. Spoon the lime juice mixture over the roasted vegetables and serve.

Nutrition Information (per serving):

Calories 203
Carbohydrate 12g
(Fiber 4g, Sugars 3g)
Fat 17g (Saturated Fat 2g)
Protein 5g

Cholesterol 0mg
Sodium 317mg
Macros: 75% Fat, 10% Protein, 15% Carbs
Net Carbs: 8g

Grilled Eggplant with Tomato Relish

SERVES 2 • PREP: 10 MINUTES • COOK: 8 MINUTES

2 tablespoons olive oil

1 teaspoon balsamic vinegar

1 garlic clove, minced

½ teaspoon fresh or dried rosemary, chopped

⅛ teaspoon kosher salt

Black pepper to taste

1 or 2 drops liquid stevia (optional)

8 ounces eggplant, cut into ½-inch-thick rounds

1 plum tomato, chopped

8 pitted kalamata olives, coarsely chopped

1 tablespoon finely chopped red onion

1. Preheat grill or grill pan to high heat.

2. In a medium bowl, whisk together the oil, vinegar, garlic, rosemary, salt, pepper, and stevia, if using. Lightly brush both sides of the eggplant slices with 1 tablespoon of the oil mixture.

3. Add the tomato, olives, and onion to the remaining oil mixture in bowl, stir until well blended, and set aside.

4. Grill the eggplant for 5 minutes on one side; turn and grill for 3 to 5 minutes or until tender.

5. Divide the eggplant slices between 2 plates. Top with equal amounts of the tomato mixture.

Nutrition Information (per serving):

Calories 199	Cholesterol 0mg
Carbohydrate 11g	Sodium 369mg
(Fiber 4g, Sugars 5g)	**Macros:** 82% Fat, 4% Protein,
Fat 18g (Saturated Fat 2.5g)	14% Carbs
Protein 2g	**Net Carbs:** 7g

Cashew-Ginger Bok Choy

SERVES 2 • TOTAL TIME: 18 MINUTES

1½ tablespoons toasted
sesame oil, divided

2 heads baby bok choy,
quartered lengthwise

2 garlic cloves, minced

2 teaspoons grated fresh
ginger

⅛ teaspoon crushed red
pepper flakes

2 teaspoons coconut
aminos

⅛ teaspoon kosher salt

2 tablespoons chopped
fresh cilantro

¼ cup chopped toasted
cashews

1. Heat 2 teaspoons of sesame oil in a large skillet over medium-high heat. Add the bok choy and cook for 4 minutes. Reduce the heat to medium, cover, and continue to cook for 3 minutes.

2. Remove the bok choy and set aside on a plate. To the skillet, add the remaining 2½ teaspoons sesame oil and the garlic, ginger, and pepper flakes; cook 15 seconds, stirring constantly. Add the coconut aminos and stir well. Add the bok choy, stir gently, and cook for 2 minutes. Sprinkle with the salt, cilantro, and cashews.

Nutrition Information (per serving):

Calories 197

Carbohydrate 9g

(Fiber 2g, Sugars 2g)

Fat 17g (Saturated Fat 2.6g)

Protein 4g

Cholesterol 0g

Sodium 308mg

Macros: 77% Fat, 8% Protein, 15% Carbs

Net Carbs: 7g

Roasted Carrots with Jalapeño-Pecan Salsa

SERVES 2 • PREP: 10 MINUTES • ROAST: 33 MINUTES

3 small or medium carrots, quartered lengthwise, and cut into 2-inch pieces

¼ cup coarsely chopped onion

1½ tablespoons toasted sesame oil, divided

½ teaspoon ground cumin

¼ teaspoon kosher salt, divided

⅛ teaspoon black pepper

⅓ cup pecans, coarsely chopped

1 jalapeño, seeded and finely chopped

1½ teaspoons balsamic vinegar

1 small garlic clove, minced

2 cups arugula

1. Preheat oven to 425°F. Line a baking sheet with foil.

2. Place the carrots and onion on the prepared baking sheet. Drizzle 1 tablespoon of the sesame oil over all and sprinkle with the cumin, ⅛ teaspoon salt, and the black pepper. Toss until well coated and spread out in a single layer.

3. Place the baking sheet on an upper (not top) oven rack and roast, stirring occasionally, 30 minutes or until the edges are lightly browned and the carrots are tender. Push the carrots and onion to one side of the baking sheet, add the pecans to the other side, and roast for 3 to 5 minutes or until lightly toasted.

4. In a small bowl, combine the pecans with the jalapeño, the remaining 1½ teaspoons sesame oil, the balsamic vinegar, garlic, and remaining ⅛ teaspoon salt.

5. Divide the arugula between two plates.

6. Using a fork, scrape up any browned bits from the baking sheet and stir into the carrots for added flavor. Serve the carrot mixture on top of the arugula and spoon the pecan mixture evenly over all.

Nutrition Information (per serving):

Calories 269

Carbohydrate 15g

(Fiber 5g, Sugars 7g)

Fat 24g (Saturated Fat 2.7g)

Protein 3g

Cholesterol 0mg

Sodium 306mg

Macros: 80% Fat, 5% Protein, 15% Carbs

Net Carbs: 10g

Eggs with Hot Pepper Oil

SERVES 1 • TOTAL TIME: 5 MINUTES

- 2 teaspoons extra-virgin olive oil
- 1 teaspoon hot pepper sauce
- 2 hard-boiled eggs, peeled and halved
- 1 teaspoon pumpkin seeds (pepitas), toasted
- 1 teaspoon chopped fresh cilantro
- Sea salt and black pepper

In a small bowl, whisk together the olive oil and pepper sauce. Drizzle over cut sides of eggs. Sprinkle with pumpkin seeds, cilantro, and a pinch each of salt and pepper.

Nutrition Information (per serving):

Calories 228
Carbohydrate 2g
(Fiber 1g, Sugars 1g)
Fat 19g (Saturated Fat 3.5g)
Protein 13g

Cholesterol 350mg
Sodium 406mg
Macros: 74% Fat, 24% Protein, 2% Carbs
Net Carbs: 1g

Creamy Herb Veggie Dip

SERVES 1 • TOTAL TIME: 5 MINUTES

- 2 tablespoons plain Greek-style vegan yogurt
- 2 tablespoons vegan chive cream cheese
- 1 tablespoon chopped fresh basil
- 1 teaspoon fresh lemon juice
- 1 tablespoon extra-virgin olive oil
- 1 tablespoon toasted pine nuts
- Black pepper
- ½ cup red bell pepper strips

1. In a small bowl, combine yogurt, cream cheese, basil, and lemon juice. Drizzle with the olive oil. Sprinkle with pine nuts and a pinch of black pepper.

2. Serve with bell pepper strips.

Nutrition Information (per serving):

Calories 325
Carbohydrate 10g
(Fiber 2g, Sugars 3g)
Fat 29g (Saturated Fat 2g)
Protein 7g

Cholesterol 0mg
Sodium 347mg
Macros: 81% Fat, 9% Protein, 10% Carbs
Net Carbs: 8g

Blueberry-Matcha Smoothie

SERVES 1 • TOTAL TIME: 5 MINUTES

½ cup full-fat coconut milk, chilled

½ cup frozen blueberries

2 tablespoons hemp protein powder

1 teaspoon matcha powder

1 teaspoon vanilla extract

½ teaspoon grated fresh ginger

Sea salt

Liquid stevia (optional)

In a blender, combine coconut milk, ¼ cup cold water, blueberries, protein powder, matcha, vanilla, ginger, and a pinch of sea salt. Cover and blend until smooth. If desired, blend in a few drops of liquid stevia.

Nutrition Information (per serving):

Calories 250	Cholesterol 0mg
Carbohydrate 17g	Sodium 190mg
(Fiber 5g, Sugars 11g)	**Macros:** 65% Fat, 17% Protein,
Fat 18g (Saturated Fat 15.5g)	18% Carbs
Protein 10g	**Net Carbs:** 12g

Coconut Lime Smoothie

SERVES 1 • TOTAL TIME: 5 MINUTES

½ cup full-fat coconut milk, chilled

2 tablespoons fresh lime juice

1 tablespoon hemp protein powder

1 teaspoon grated fresh ginger

1 teaspoon vanilla extract

Sea salt

Liquid stevia (optional)

In a blender, combine coconut milk, ½ cup cold water, lime juice, protein powder, ginger, vanilla, and a pinch of sea salt. Cover and blend until smooth. If desired, blend in a few drops of liquid stevia.

Nutrition Information (per serving):

Calories 202	Cholesterol 0mg
Carbohydrate 9g	Sodium 187mg
(Fiber 2g, Sugars 4g)	**Macros:** 77% Fat, 9% Protein,
Fat 17g (Saturated Fat 15g)	14% Carbs
Protein 5g	**Net Carbs:** 7g

Strawberry-Spirulina Smoothie

SERVES 1 • TOTAL TIME: 5 MINUTES

½ cup frozen strawberries

½ small avocado, pitted and peeled

¾ cup unsweetened almond milk

1 tablespoon hemp protein powder

1½ teaspoons spirulina powder

1 teaspoon vanilla extract

Sea salt

Liquid stevia (optional)

In a blender, combine strawberries, avocado, almond milk, protein powder, spirulina powder, vanilla, and a pinch of sea salt. Blend until smooth. If desired, blend in a few drops of liquid stevia.

Nutrition Information (per serving):

Calories 198

Carbohydrate 19g

(Fiber 8g, Sugars 5g)

Fat 13g (Saturated Fat 1.5g)

Protein 9g

Cholesterol 0mg

Sodium 346mg

Macros: 58% Fat, 19% Protein, 23% Carbs

Net Carbs: 11g

Pineapple Smoothie

SERVES 1 • TOTAL TIME: 5 MINUTES

½ cup chopped fresh pineapple

½ cup unsweetened almond milk

½ cup full-fat coconut milk

2 tablespoons hemp protein powder

1 tablespoon fresh lime juice

1 teaspoon vanilla extract

Sea salt

Liquid stevia (optional)

In a blender, combine pineapple, almond milk, coconut milk, protein powder, lime juice, vanilla, and a pinch of sea salt. Cover and blend until smooth. If desired, blend in a few drops of liquid stevia.

Nutrition Information (per serving):

Calories 277

Carbohydrate 21g

(Fiber 5g, Sugars 12g)

Fat 20g (Saturated Fat 15.5g)

Protein 9g

Cholesterol 0mg

Sodium 280mg

Macros: 65% Fat, 17% Protein, 18% Carbs

Net Carbs: 16g

Salted Dark Chocolate–Almond Bark

SERVES 1 • **TOTAL TIME: 20 MINUTES**

1 ounce unsweetened chocolate

Liquid stevia (optional)

1 tablespoon finely chopped almonds

Sea salt

1. In a small microwave-safe bowl, microwave chocolate on low in 15-second intervals, stopping to stir, until melted and smooth. If desired, stir in a few drops of liquid stevia.

2. Spread in an even layer on a piece of parchment paper. Sprinkle with almonds and a pinch of sea salt.

3. Refrigerate 15 minutes or until set. Break into pieces.

Nutrition Information (per serving):

Calories 185

Carbohydrate 9g

(Fiber 7g, Sugars 0g)

Fat 17g (Saturated Fat 9.5g)

Protein 5g

Cholesterol 0mg

Sodium 148mg

Macros: 83% Fat, 11% Protein, 6% Carbs

Net Carbs: 2g

Spicy Almond Butter Dip

SERVES 1 • TOTAL TIME: 5 MINUTES

2 tablespoons almond butter

1½ tablespoons unsweetened almond milk

½ teaspoon fresh lemon juice

½ teaspoon grated fresh ginger

Sea salt

Smoked paprika

Cayenne pepper

Liquid stevia (optional)

In a small bowl, stir together the almond butter, almond milk, lemon juice, ginger, and a pinch each of salt, paprika, and cayenne. If desired, add a few drops of liquid stevia.

Nutrition Information (per serving):

Calories 194

Carbohydrate 7g

(Fiber 3g, Sugars 2g)

Fat 17g (Saturated Fat 1.5g)

Protein 6g

Cholesterol 0mg

Sodium 165mg

Macros: 80% Fat, 13% Protein, 7% Carbs

Net Carbs: 4g

Yogurt Bowls with Cinnamon Chia Berries

SERVES 2 • PREP: 10 MINUTES • CHILL: 2 HOURS

½ cup sliced almonds

2 tablespoons unsweetened dried coconut flakes

⅓ cup frozen raspberries

⅓ cup frozen blueberries

2 teaspoons chia seeds

2 to 4 drops liquid stevia, or to taste

¼ to ½ teaspoon ground cinnamon, or to taste

½ teaspoon vanilla extract

1½ cups unsweetened plain vegan yogurt

1. Heat a medium skillet over medium-high heat until hot. Add the almonds and cook for 3 minutes or until beginning to brown, stirring frequently. Add the coconut and cook for 1 minute or until beginning to brown, stirring frequently. Remove from heat and set aside. When cooled, you may store in an airtight container until needed.

2. In a small bowl, combine the frozen raspberries, blueberries, chia seeds, stevia, cinnamon, and vanilla. Cover and refrigerate overnight or at least 2 hours.

3. To serve, divide the yogurt between 2 bowls. Stir the berry mixture and spoon equal amounts on the yogurt. Crumble the almond mixture and sprinkle it on top of the berry sauce.

Nutrition Information (per serving):

Calories 356

Carbohydrate 22g

(Fiber 9g, Sugars 5g)

Fat 29g (Saturated Fat 4.6g)

Protein 12g

Cholesterol 11mg

Sodium 14mg

Macros: 72% Fat, 13% Protein, 15% Carbs

Net Carbs: 13g

Fruit Yogurt Cup

SERVES 1 • **TOTAL TIME: 5 MINUTES**

½ cup plain Greek-style
vegan yogurt
Liquid stevia (optional)
¼ cup blackberries
¼ cup chopped toasted
almonds

Place yogurt in a small bowl. If desired, stir in a few drops of liquid stevia. Top with blackberries and almonds.

Nutrition Information (per serving):

Calories 346
Carbohydrate 15g
(Fiber 6g, Sugars 4g)
Fat 27g (Saturated Fat 1.5g)
Protein 16g

Cholesterol 0mg
Sodium 5mg
Macros: 70% Fat, 19% Protein,
11% Carbs
Net Carbs: 9g

Avocado "Toasts"

SERVES 1 • **TIME: 5 MINUTES**

½ small avocado, pitted
and peeled
Lemon wedge
Sea salt
8 sea salt flaxseed
crackers
Crushed red pepper
flakes
1 radish, thinly sliced

In a small bowl, combine avocado, juice of lemon wedge, and a pinch of sea salt. Mash until desired consistency. Spread evenly over the crackers. Sprinkle with pepper flakes. Top with sliced radish.

Nutrition Information (per serving):

Calories 210
Carbohydrate 14g
(Fiber 12g, Sugars 1g)
Fat 19g (Saturated Fat 2.5g)
Protein 6g

Cholesterol 0mg
Sodium 362mg
Macros: 84% Fat, 12% Protein,
5% Carbs
Net Carbs: 2g

Crackers with Chive Cheese Spread

SERVES 1 • TOTAL TIME: 5 MINUTES

2 tablespoons chive vegan cream cheese

8 sea salt flaxseed crackers

1 tablespoon extra-virgin olive oil

Spread the cream cheese evenly over the crackers. Drizzle evenly with the olive oil.

Nutrition Information (per serving):

Calories 336

Carbohydrate 11g

(Fiber 7g, Sugars 0g)

Fat 32g (Saturated Fat 3g)

Protein 8g

Cholesterol 0mg

Sodium 330mg

Macros: 85% Fat, 10% Protein, 5% Carbs

Net Carbs: 4g

Cocoa-Covered Almond Fat Bombs

SERVES 1 • TOTAL TIME: 35 MINUTES

1 tablespoon almond butter

1½ teaspoons coconut oil, melted

¼ teaspoon vanilla extract

Sea salt

Liquid stevia (optional)

1 teaspoon unsweetened cocoa

1. In a small bowl, combine the almond butter, coconut oil, vanilla, and a pinch of salt. If desired, stir in a drop of stevia. Cover and refrigerate for 30 to 40 minutes.

2. Shape into two balls. Roll in unsweetened cocoa to coat.

Nutrition Information (per serving):

Calories 257

Carbohydrate 7g

(Fiber 4g, Sugars 2g)

Fat 24g (Saturated Fat 7.5g)

Protein 6g

Cholesterol 0mg

Sodium 145mg

Macros: 85% Fat, 10% Protein, 5% Carbs

Net Carbs: 3g

Marinated Cheese and Olives with Melon and Cucumber

SERVES 1 • TOTAL TIME: 5 MINUTES

1½ ounces fresh-style vegan mozzarella cheese, cubed

6 pitted kalamata olives

1½ tablespoons extra-virgin olive oil

¼ teaspoon grated lemon zest

¼ teaspoon chopped fresh rosemary

Sea salt and black pepper

¼ cup sliced cucumber

¼ cup cubed honeydew melon

1. In a medium bowl, combine the cheese, olives, olive oil, lemon zest, rosemary, and a pinch each of salt and pepper. Cover and chill until ready to serve.

2. Serve with cucumber and melon.

Nutrition Information (per serving):

Calories 371

Carbohydrate 10g

(Fiber 1g, Sugars 4g)

Fat 36g (Saturated Fat 10g)

Protein 1g

Cholesterol 0mg

Sodium 616mg

Macros: 88% Fat, 2% Protein, 10% Carbs

Net Carbs: 9g

Lox-Stuffed Cucumber

SERVES 1 • TOTAL TIME: 5 MINUTES

1 hard-boiled egg, peeled and chopped

2 teaspoons avocado oil mayonnaise

1 teaspoon chopped fresh dill

½ teaspoon Dijon mustard

½ teaspoon chopped capers

Sea salt and black pepper

1 small cucumber, cut in half lengthwise and seeded

1 ounce lox or smoked salmon, torn into small pieces

In a small bowl, combine egg, mayonnaise, dill, mustard, capers, and a pinch each of salt and pepper. Spoon into cucumber halves. Top with salmon.

Nutrition Information (per serving):

Calories 180

Carbohydrate 3g

(Fiber 1g, Sugars 2g)

Fat 13g (Saturated Fat 2g)

Protein 12g

Cholesterol 192mg

Sodium 401mg

Macros: 67% Fat, 29% Protein, 4% Carbs

Net Carbs: 2g

How to Pressure Cook Dried Beans

1 pound dried beans or chickpeas, sorted, rinsed, and drained (yields 2½ to 3¼ cups of cooked beans, depending on the type of bean)

1. Add beans and 8 cups water to the pressure cooker pot. Lock the lid in place and close the seal valve. Press the Manual button to set the cook time for time recommended below. When the cook time ends, use a natural pressure release.

2. When the valve drops, carefully remove the lid. Drain the beans in a colander.

Pinto Beans: 25 Minutes on High Pressure

Black Beans: 30 Minutes on High Pressure

Navy Beans: 30 Minutes on High Pressure

Great Northern Beans: 35 Minutes on High Pressure

Kidney Beans: 35 Minutes on High Pressure

Chickpeas: 40 Minutes on High Pressure

Makes 6 cups cooked beans or chickpeas. Store the cooled beans in smaller quantities in freezer bags. Freezes for up to 3 months (or keeps for 5 days in the refrigerator). You may add a small amount of liquid to keep them moist, but remember to drain before using.

Note: You don't need to soak beans before cooking in the pressure cooker, but if soaking is desired, cook for 10 minutes less under pressure.

Acknowledgments

Amber, Solomon, and Shiloh: I love you so freaking much. Thank you for being my center and my safe place.

My team: Andrea, Yvette, Emily, Janice, Megan, Brinna, Hollie, and Maddy: You are part of my family and my closest friends. Thank you for your consistent devotion, diligence, and compassion for our patients and for one another.

My patients around the world: Thank you for letting me be a part of your sacred journey into wellness. I do not take that responsibility lightly. Serving you is truly an honor.

Heather, Diana, Michele, and everyone at Rodale and Waterbury: You are the best team I could have dreamed of. Thank you for always listening to my vision and doing everything to help it come to life.

Gretchen: Thank you for your friendship and putting your heart into this book with me.

Gwyneth, Elise, Kiki, and my goop family: I am immensely grateful for you. Thank you for your years of friendship and for championing me.

Dr. Alejandro Junger, Melissa Urban, Dr. Terry Wahls, and Dr. Josh Axe: Thank you for being my mentors, heroes, and good friends in this space of wellness.

Finally, thank you to everyone in the functional medicine and wellness world: Continue being a light.

Notes

CHAPTER 1

1   Byrne NM, Sainsbury A, King NA, et al. Intermittent energy restriction improves weight loss efficiency in obese men; the matador study. *Int J Obes* (Lond). 2018;42(2):129–138. doi:10.1038/ijo.2017.206.

2   Baker DB & Keramidas N. The psychology of hunger. *Monitor on Psychology*. 2013 Oct;44(9). http://www.apa.org/monitor/2013/10/hunger.

3   Carter S, Clifton PM, Keogh JB. The effects of intermittent compared to continuous energy restriction on glycaemic control in type 2 diabetes: a pragmatic pilot trial. *Diabetes Res Clin Pract*. 2016;122:106–112. doi:10.1016/j.diabres.2016.10.010.

4   Kahleova H, Belinova L, Malinska H, et al. Eating two larger meals a day (breakfast and lunch) is more effective than six smaller meals in a reduced-energy regimen for patients with type 2 diabetes: a randomised crossover study [published correction appears in *Diabetologia*. 2015 Jan;58(1):205]. *Diabetologia*. 2014;57(8):1552–1560. doi:10.1007/s00125-014-3253-5.

5   Chapelot D. The role of snacking in energy balance: a biobehavioral approach. *J Nutr*. 2011;141(1):158–162. doi:10.3945/jn.109.114330.

6   Ribeiro AG, Costa MJ, Faintuch J, Dias MC. A higher meal frequency may be associated with diminished weight loss after bariatric surgery. *Clinics* (Sao Paulo). 2009;64(11):1053–1058. doi:10.1590/S1807-59322009001100004.

7   Fildes A, Charlton J, Rudisill C, et al. Probability of an obese person attaining normal body weight: cohort study using electronic health records. *Am J Public Health*. 2015;105(9):e54–e59. doi:10.2105/AJPH.2015.302773.

8   Harvie MN, Pegington M, Mattson MP, et al. The effects of intermittent or continuous energy restriction on weight loss and metabolic disease

risk markers: a randomized trial in young overweight women. *Int J Obes (Lond).* 2011;35(5):714–727. doi:10.1038/ijo.2010.171.

9 de Cabo, R., & Mattson, M. P. Effects of intermittent fasting on health, aging, and disease. *N Engl J Med.* 2019;381(26): 2541–2551. https://doi.org/10.1056/nejmra1905136.

10 Fasting. (n.d.). Retrieved September 2, 2020, from *Encyclopedia Britannica* website: https://www.britannica.com/topic/fasting.

11 Penny F. Notes on a thirty days' fast. *Br Med.* 1909 Jun;1(2528):1414–16. doi: 10.1136/bmj.1.2528.1414.

12 Kim JM. Ketogenic diet: Old treatment, new beginning. *Clin Neurophysiol Pract.* 2017;2:161–2. Published 2017 Jul 24. doi:10.1016/j.cnp.2017.07.001; https://www.ncbi.nlm.nih.gov/pmc/articles/PMC6123870/.

13 Gilliland IC. Total fasting in the treatment of obesity. *Postgrad Med J.* 1968;44(507):58-61. doi:10.1136/pgmj.44.507.58; https://pmj.bmj.com/content/postgradmedj/44/507/58.full.pdf.

14 Hartman AL, Rubenstein JE, Kossoff EH. Intermittent fasting: a "new" historical strategy for controlling seizures? *Epilepsy Res.* 2013;104(3):275–279. doi:10.1016/j.eplepsyres.2012.10.011.

15 Cordain L, Eaton SB, Sebastian A, et al. Origins and evolution of the western diet: health implications for the 21st century. *Am J Clin Nut.* 2005;81(2):341–54. doi:10.1093/ajcn.81.2.341.

16 Mattson MP. An evolutionary perspective on why food overconsumption impairs cognition. *Trends Cogn Sci.* 2019;23(3):200–12. doi:10.1016/j.tics.2019.01.003.

CHAPTER 2

1 Kallus SJ, Brandt LJ. The intestinal microbiota and obesity. *J Clin Gas-*troenterol. 2012;46(1):16–24. doi:10.1097/MCG.0b013e31823711fd.

2 Suez J, Korem T, Zeevi D, et al. Artificial sweeteners induce glucose intolerance by altering the gut microbiota. *Nature.* 2014;514(7521):181–186. doi:10.1038/nature13793.

3 Wang H, Lu Y, Yan Y, et al. Promising treatment for type 2 diabetes: fecal microbiota transplantation reverses insulin resistance and impaired islets. *Front Cell Infect Microbiol.* 2020;9:455. Published 2020 Jan 17. doi:10.3389/fcimb.2019.00455.

4 Alcock J, Maley CC, Aktipis CA. Is eating behavior manipulated by the gastrointestinal microbiota? Evolutionary pressures and potential mechanisms. *Bioessays.* 2014;36(10):940–49. doi:10.1002/bies.201400071.

5 Rousseaux C, Thuru X, Gelot A, et al. *Lactobacillus acidophilus* modulates intestinal pain and induces opioid and cannabinoid receptors. *Nat Med.* 2007;13(1):35–7. doi:10.1038/nm1521.

6 Perry RJ, Wang Y, Cline GW, et al. Leptin mediates a glucose-fatty acid cycle to maintain glucose homeostasis in starvation. *Cell.* 2018;172(1-2):234-248.e17. doi:10.1016/j.cell.2017.12.001.

7 Zhou Y, Rui L. Leptin signaling and leptin resistance. *Front Med.* 2013;7(2):207–22. doi:10.1007/s11684-013-0263-5.

8 Chetty S, Friedman AR, Taravosh-Lahn K, et al. Stress and glucocorticoids promote oligodendrogenesis in the adult hippocampus. *Mol Psychiatry.* 2014;19(12):1275–83. doi:10.1038/mp.2013.190.

9 Workplace stressors & health outcomes: Health policy for the workplace | Behavioral Science & Policy Association. Accessed September 2, 2020. https://behavioralpolicy.org/articles/workplace-stressors-health-outcomes-health-policy-for-the-workplace/.

10 Pillai V, Roth T, Mullins HM, Drake CL. Moderators and mediators of the relationship between stress and insomnia: stressor chronicity, cognitive intrusion, and coping. *Sleep.* 2014;37(7):1199–1208. Published 2014 Jul 1. doi:10.5665/sleep.3838.

11 Wang HX, Wahlberg M, Karp A, et al. Psychosocial stress at work is associated with increased dementia risk in late life. *Alzheimers Dement.* 2012;8(2):114–20. doi:10.1016/j.jalz.2011.03.001.

12 Sinha R, Jastreboff AM. Stress as a common risk factor for obesity and addiction. *Biol Psychiatry.* 2013;73(9):827-835. doi:10.1016/j.biopsych.2013.01.032.

13 Konturek PC, Brzozowski T, Konturek SJ. Stress and the gut: pathophysiology, clinical consequences, diagnostic approach and treatment options. *J Physiol Pharmacol.* 2011;62(6):591-99.

14 Cohen S, Janicki-Deverts D, Doyle WJ, et al. Chronic stress, glucocorticoid receptor resistance, inflammation, and disease risk. *Proc Natl Acad Sci USA.* 2012;109(16):5995-99. doi:10.1073/pnas.1118355109.

15 Burcelin R, Garidou L, Pomié C. Immuno-microbiota cross and talk: the new paradigm of metabolic diseases. *Semin Immunol.* 2012;24(1):67–74. doi:10.1016/j.smim.2011.11.011.

16 Ohman MK, Wright AP, Wickenheiser KJ, et al. Visceral adipose tissue and atherosclerosis. *Curr Vasc Pharmacol.* 2009;7(2):169-179. doi:10.2174/157016109787455680.

17 Jung SH, Ha KH, Kim DJ. Visceral fat mass has stronger associations with diabetes and prediabetes than other anthropometric obesity indicators among Korean adults. *Yonsei Med J.* 2016;57(3):674-680. doi:10.3349/ymj.2016.57.3.674.

CHAPTER 3

1   Mary Poppins was an Enabler. UC Health–UC San Diego. Published October 27, 2017. Accessed September 4, 2020. https://health.ucsd.edu/news/features/pages/2017-10-27-listicle-mary-poppins-was-an-enabler.aspx#:~:text=Today%2C%20Americans%20consume%2C%20on%20average,mostly%20sugar%2Dfree%201822%20predecessors.

2   de Cabo R, Mattson MP. Effects of intermittent fasting on health, aging, and disease [published correction appears in N Engl J Med. 2020 Jan 16;382(3):298] [published correction appears in N Engl J Med. 2020 Mar 5;382(10):978]. N Engl J Med. 2019;381(26):2541–51. doi:10.1056/NEJMra1905136.

3   de Cabo R, Mattson MP. Effects of intermittent fasting on health, aging, and disease [published correction appears in N Engl J Med. 2020 Jan 16;382(3):298] [published correction appears in N Engl J Med. 2020 Mar 5;382(10):978]. N Engl J Med. 2019;381(26):2541–51. doi:10.1056/NEJMra1905136.

4   Youm YH, Nguyen KY, Grant RW, et al. The ketone metabolite β-hydroxybutyrate blocks NLRP3 inflammasome-mediated inflammatory disease. Nat Med. 2015;21(3):263–69. doi:10.1038/nm.3804.

5   Mayor A. The Poison King: The Life and Legend of Mithradates, Rome's Deadliest Enemy. Princeton University Press; Princeton, NJ, USA: 2010. p. 242.

6   Glick D, Barth S, Macleod KF. Autophagy: cellular and molecular mechanisms. J Pathol. 2010;221(1):3–12. doi:10.1002/path.2697.

7   Mattson MP, Arumugam TV. Hallmarks of brain aging: adaptive and pathological modification by metabolic states. Cell Metab.

8   Xihang Chen, Yunfan He, Feng Lu. Autophagy in stem cell biology: a perspective on stem cell self-renewal and differentiation. Stem Cells Int. 2018; 2018: 9131397.

9   Levine B, Kroemer G. Autophagy in the pathogenesis of disease. Cell. 2008;132(1):27–42. doi:10.1016/j.cell.2007.12.018.

10   Goodrick CL, Ingram DK, Reynolds MA, et al. Effects of intermittent feeding upon growth and life span in rats. Gerontology. 1982;28(4):233–41. doi:10.1159/000212538.

11   Xie K, Neff F, Markert A, et al. Every-other-day feeding extends lifespan but fails to delay many symptoms of aging in mice. Nat Commun. 2017;8(1):155. Published 2017 Jul 24. doi:10.1038/s41467-017-00178-3; https://www.ncbi.nlm.nih.gov/pmc/articles/PMC5537224/.

12   Elamin M, Ruskin DN, Masino SA, Sacchetti P. Ketogenic diet modulates NAD+-dependent enzymes and reduces DNA damage in hippocampus. Front Cell Neurosci. 2018;12:263. Published 2018 Aug 30. doi:10.3389/fncel.2018.00263.

13   Imai S, Guarente L. NAD+ and sirtuins in aging and disease. Trends Cell Biol. 2014;24(8):464–71. doi:10.1016/j.tcb.2014.04.002.

14   Grabowska W, Sikora E, Bielak-Zmijewska A. Sirtuins, a promising target in slowing down the ageing process. Biogerontology. 2017;18(4):447–76. doi:10.1007/s10522-017-9685-9.

15   Lee JY, Kennedy BK, Liao CY. Mechanistic target of rapamycin signaling in mouse models of accelerated aging. J Gerontol A Biol Sci Med Sci. 2020;75(1):64–72. doi:10.1093/gerona/glz059.

16   Roth GS, Ingram DK. Manipulation of health span and function by

dietary caloric restriction mimetics. Ann N Y Acad Sci. 2016;1363:5–10. doi:10.1111/nyas.12834.

17   Mattson MP, Arumugam TV. Hallmarks of brain aging: adaptive and pathological modification by metabolic states. Cell Metab. 2018;27(6):1176–1199. doi:10.1016/j.cmet.2018.05.011.

18   Jordan S, Tung N, Casanova-Acebes M, et al. Dietary intake regulates the circulating inflammatory monocyte pool. Cell. 2019;178(5):1102–14.e17. doi:10.1016/j.cell.2019.07.050.

19   Chaix A, Zarrinpar A, Miu P, Panda S. Time-restricted feeding is a preventative and therapeutic intervention against diverse nutritional challenges. Cell Metab. 2014;20(6):991–1005. doi:10.1016/j.cmet.2014.11.001.

20   Johnson JB, Summer W, Cutler RG, et al. Alternate day calorie restriction improves clinical findings and reduces markers of oxidative stress and inflammation in overweight adults with moderate asthma [published correction appears in Free Radic Biol Med. 2007 Nov 1;43(9):1348. Tellejohan, Richard [corrected to Telljohann, Richard]]. Free Radic Biol Med. 2007;42(5):665–74. doi:10.1016/j.freeradbiomed.2006.12.005.

21   Gabel K, Hoddy KK, Haggerty N, et al. Effects of 8-hour time restricted feeding on body weight and metabolic disease risk factors in obese adults: A pilot study. Nutr Healthy Aging. 2018 Jun 15;4(4):345–53. doi:10.3233/NHA-170036.

22   Seimon RV, Roekenes JA, Zibellini J, et al. Do intermittent diets provide physiological benefits over continuous diets for weight loss? A systematic review of clinical trials. Mol Cell Endocrinol. 2015;418 Pt 2:153–72. doi:10.1016/j.mce.2015.09.014.

23   Wilkinson MJ, Manoogian ENC, Zadourian A, et al. Ten-hour time-

restricted eating reduces weight, blood pressure, and atherogenic lipids in patients with metabolic syndrome. *Cell Metab.* 2020;31(1):92–104.e5. doi:10.1016/j.cmet.2019.11.004.

24 Sutton EF, Beyl R, Early KS, et al. Early time-restricted feeding improves insulin sensitivity, blood pressure, and oxidative stress even without weight loss in men with prediabetes. *Cell Metab.* 2018;27(6):1212–21.e3. doi:10.1016/j.cmet.2018.04.010.

25 Intermountain Medical Center. 2011 May 20. Routine periodic fasting is good for your health, and your heart, study suggests. *ScienceDaily.* Retrieved September 1, 2020 from www.sciencedaily.com/releases/2011/04/110403090259.htm.

26 Moro T, Tinsley G, Bianco A, et al. Effects of eight weeks of time-restricted feeding (16/8) on basal metabolism, maximal strength, body composition, inflammation, and cardiovascular risk factors in resistance-trained males. *J Transl Med.* 2016 Oct 13;14(1):290. doi:10.1186/s12967-016-1044-0.

CHAPTER 4

1 Arble DM, Ramsey KM, Bass J, Turek FW. Circadian disruption and metabolic disease: findings from animal models. *Best Pract Res Clin Endocrinol Metab.* 2010;24(5):785–800. doi:10.1016/j.beem.2010.08.003.

2 Loh DH, Jami SA, Flores RE, et al. Misaligned feeding impairs memories. *Elife.* 2015 Dec 10;4:e09460. doi:10.7554/eLife.09460.

CHAPTER 5

1 McClernon FJ, Yancy WS Jr, Eberstein JA, et al. The effects of a low-carbohydrate ketogenic diet and a low-fat diet on mood, hunger, and other self-reported symptoms. *Obesity* (Silver Spring). 2007;15(1):182–87. doi:10.1038/oby.2007.516.

2 Jakubowicz D, Froy O, Wainstein J, Boaz M. Meal timing and composition influence ghrelin levels, appetite scores and weight loss maintenance in overweight and obese adults [published correction appears in *Steroids.* 2012 Jul;77(8–9):887–9]. *Steroids.* 2012;77(4):323–31. doi:10.1016/j.steroids.2011.12.006.

3 Ravussin E, Beyl RA, Poggiogalle E, Hsia DS, Peterson CM. Early time-restricted feeding reduces appetite and increases fat oxidation but does not affect energy expenditure in humans. *Obesity* (Silver Spring). 2019;27(8):1244–54. doi:10.1002/oby.22518.

4 Mysels DJ, Sullivan MA. The relationship between opioid and sugar intake: review of evidence and clinical applications. *J Opioid Manag.* 2010;6(6):445–52. doi:10.5055/jom.2010.0043.

5 Bray GA. Is sugar addictive?. *Diabetes.* 2016;65(7):1797–99. doi:10.2337/dbi16-0022.

6 Castro AI, Gomez-Arbelaez D, Crujeiras AB, et al. Effect of a very low-calorie ketogenic diet on food and alcohol cravings, physical and sexual activity, sleep disturbances, and quality of life in obese patients. *Nutrients.* 2018 Sep 21;10(10):1348. doi:10.3390/nu10101348.

7 David LA, Maurice CF, Carmody RN, et al. Diet rapidly and reproducibly alters the human gut microbiome. *Nature.* 2014;505(7484):559–63. doi:10.1038/nature12820.

8 Cani PD, Amar J, Iglesias MA, et al. Metabolic endotoxemia initiates obesity and insulin resistance. *Diabetes.* 2007;56(7):1761–72. doi:10.2337/db06-1491.

9 Kanazawa M, Fukudo S. Effects of fasting therapy on irritable bowel syndrome. *Int J Behav Med.* 2006;13(3):214–20. doi:10.1207/s15327558ijbm1303_4.

10 Aksungar FB, Topkaya AE, Akyildiz M. Interleukin-6, C-reactive protein and biochemical parameters during prolonged intermittent fasting. *Ann Nutr Metab.* 2007;51(1):88–95. doi:10.1159/000100954.

CHAPTER 6

1 Patterson RE, Sears DD. Metabolic effects of intermittent fasting. *Annu Rev Nutr.* 2017;37:371–93. doi:10.1146/annurev-nutr-071816-064634.

2 Patterson RE, Laughlin GA, LaCroix AZ, et al. Intermittent fasting and human metabolic health. *J Acad Nutr Diet.* 2015;115(8):1203–12. doi:10.1016/j.jand.2015.02.018.

3 Chen IJ, Liu CY, Chiu JP, Hsu CH. Therapeutic effect of high-dose green tea extract on weight reduction: a randomized, double-blind, placebo-controlled clinical trial. *Clin Nutr.* 2016;35(3):592–99. doi:10.1016/j.clnu.2015.05.003.

4 Rothschild J, Hoddy KK, Jambazian P, Varady KA. Time-restricted feeding and risk of metabolic disease: a review of human and animal studies. *Nutr Rev.* 2014;72(5):308–18. doi:10.1111/nure.12104.

5 Fasting reduces cholesterol levels in prediabetic people over extended period of time, new research finds. *ScienceDaily.* https://www.sciencedaily.com/releases/2014/06/140614150142.htm. Accessed September 3, 2020.

6 Collier R. Intermittent fasting: the next big weight loss fad. *CMAJ.* 2013;185(8):E321–E322. doi:10.1503/cmaj.109-4437.

7 Diabetes UK Professional Conference (DUPC) 2019: Talk entitled Intermittent fasting: weight loss and beyond. Presented March 7, 2019.

8 Harvie M, Wright C, Pegington M, et al. The effect of intermittent energy and carbohydrate restriction v. daily energy restriction on weight loss

and metabolic disease risk markers in overweight women. *Br J Nutr.* 2013;110(8):1534–47. doi:10.1017/S0007114513000792.

9   Sutton EF, Beyl R, Early KS, et al. Early time-restricted feeding improves insulin sensitivity, blood pressure, and oxidative stress even without weight loss in men with prediabetes. *Cell Metab.* 2018;27(6):1212–21.e3. doi:10.1016/j.cmet.2018.04.010.

10   Heilbronn LK, Smith SR, Martin CK, et al. Alternate-day fasting in nonobese subjects: effects on body weight, body composition, and energy metabolism. *Am J Clin Nutr.* 2005;81(1):69–73. doi:10.1093/ajcn/81.1.69.

11   Gershuni VM, Yan SL, Medici V. Nutritional ketosis for weight management and reversal of metabolic syndrome. *Curr Nutr Rep.* 2018;7(3):97–106. doi:10.1007/s13668-018-0235-0.

12   Furmli S, Elmasry R, Ramos M, Fung J. Therapeutic use of intermittent fasting for people with type 2 diabetes as an alternative to insulin. *BMJ Case Rep.* 2018 Oct 9;2018:bcr2017221854. doi:10.1136/bcr-2017-221854.

13   Jamshed H, Beyl RA, Della Manna DL, et al. Early time-restricted feeding improves 24-hour glucose levels and affects markers of the circadian clock, aging, and autophagy in humans. *Nutrients.* 2019;11(6):1234. Published 2019 May 30. doi:10.3390/nu11061234.

14   Anton SD, Moehl K, Donahoo WT, et al. Flipping the metabolic switch: understanding and applying the health benefits of fasting. *Obesity* (Silver Spring). 2018;26(2):254–68. doi:10.1002/oby.22065.

15   Hasan-Olive MM, Lauritzen KH, Ali M, Rasmussen LJ, et al. A ketogenic diet improves mitochondrial biogenesis and bioenergetics via the PGC1α-SIRT3-UCP2 axis. *Neurochem Res.* 2019;44(1):22–37. doi:10.1007/s11064-018-2588-6.

16   Muoio DM. Metabolic inflexibility: when mitochondrial indecision leads to metabolic gridlock. *Cell.* 2014;159(6):1253–62. doi:10.1016/j.cell.2014.11.034.

17   Morris G, Maes M. Increased nuclear factor-κB and loss of p53 are key mechanisms in myalgic encephalomyelitis/chronic fatigue syndrome (ME/CFS). Med *Hypotheses.* 2012;79(5):607–13. doi:10.1016/j.mehy.2012.07.034.

18   Li B, Zhao J, Lv J, et al. Additive antidepressant-like effects of fasting with imipramine via modulation of 5-HT2 receptors in the mice. *Prog Neuropsychopharmacol Biol Psychiatry.* 2014;48:199–206. doi:10.1016/j.pnpbp.2013.08.015.

19   Alirezaei M, Kemball CC, Flynn CT, et al. Short-term fasting induces profound neuronal autophagy. *Autophagy.* 2010;6(6):702–10. doi:10.4161/auto.6.6.12376.

20   Fond G, Macgregor A, Leboyer M, Michalsen A. Fasting in mood disorders: neurobiology and effectiveness: a review of the literature. *Psychiatry Res.* 2013;209(3):253–58. doi:10.1016/j.psychres.2012.12.018.

CHAPTER 7

1   Collier R. Intermittent fasting: the science of going without. *CMAJ.* 2013;185(9):E363–E364. doi:10.1503/cmaj.109-4451.

2   Nakamura T, Furuhashi M, Li P, et al. Double-stranded RNA-dependent protein kinase links pathogen sensing with stress and metabolic homeostasis. *Cell.* 2010;140(3):338–48. doi:10.1016/j.cell.2010.01.001.

3   Nosaka N, Suzuki Y, Nagatoishi A, et al. Effect of ingestion of medium-chain triacylglycerols on moderate- and high-intensity exercise in recreational athletes. *J Nutr Sci Vitaminol* (Tokyo). 2009;55(2):120–25. doi:10.3177/jnsv.55.120.

4   de Cabo R, Mattson MP. Effects of intermittent fasting on health, aging, and disease [published correction appears in *N Engl J Med.* 2020 Jan 16;382(3):298] [published correction appears in *N Engl J Med.* 2020 Mar 5;382(10):978]. *N Engl J Med.* 2019;381(26):2541–51. doi:10.1056/NEJMra1905136.

5   Choi IY, Piccio L, Childress P, et al. A diet mimicking fasting promotes regeneration and reduces autoimmunity and multiple sclerosis symptoms. *Cell Rep.* 2016;15(10):2136–46. doi:10.1016/j.celrep.2016.05.009.

6   Cignarella F, Cantoni C, Ghezzi L, et al. Intermittent fasting confers protection in CNS autoimmunity by altering the gut microbiota. *Cell Metab.* 2018;27(6):1222–35.e6. doi:10.1016/j.cmet.2018.05.006.

7   Jordan S, Tung N, Casanova-Acebes M, et al. Dietary intake regulates the circulating inflammatory monocyte pool. *Cell.* 2019;178(5):1102–14.e17. doi:10.1016/j.cell.2019.07.050.

8   Marinac CR, Nelson SH, Breen CI, et al. Prolonged nightly fasting and breast cancer prognosis. *JAMA Oncol.* 2016;2(8):1049–55. doi:10.1001/jamaoncol.2016.0164.

9   de Cabo R, Mattson MP. Effects of intermittent fasting on health, aging, and disease [published correction appears in *N Engl J Med.* 2020 Jan 16;382(3):298] [published correction appears in *N Engl J Med.* 2020 Mar 5;382(10):978]. *N Engl J Med.* 2019;381(26):2541–51. doi:10.1056/NEJMra1905136.

10   de Groot S, Pijl H, van der Hoeven JJM, Kroep JR. Effects of short-term fasting on cancer treatment. *J Exp Clin Cancer Res.* 2019 May 22;38(1):209. doi:10.1186/s13046-019-1189-9.

11 Raffaghello L, Safdie F, Bianchi G, et al. Fasting and differential chemotherapy protection in patients. *Cell Cycle*. 2010;9(22):4474–76. doi:10.4161/cc.9.22.13954.

12 Wolburg H, Lippoldt A. Tight junctions of the blood-brain barrier: development, composition and regulation. *Vascul Pharmacol*. 2002;38(6):323–37. doi:10.1016/s1537-1891(02)00200-8.

13 Dudek KA, Dion-Albert L, Lebel M, et al. Molecular adaptations of the blood-brain barrier promote stress resilience vs. depression. *Proc Natl Acad Sci U S A*. 2020;117(6):3326–36. doi:10.1073/pnas.1914655117.

14 Lee CH, Giuliani F. The role of inflammation in depression and fatigue. *Front Immunol*. 2019 Jul 19;10:1696. doi:10.3389/fimmu.2019.01696.

15 Schrott LM, Crnic LS. Increased anxiety behaviors in autoimmune mice. *Behav Neurosci*. 1996;110(3):492–502. doi:10.1037//0735-7044.110.3.492.

16 Faris MA, Kacimi S, Al-Kurd RA, et al. Intermittent fasting during Ramadan attenuates proinflammatory cytokines and immune cells in healthy subjects. *Nutr Res*. 2012;32(12):947–55. doi:10.1016/j.nutres.2012.06.021.

CHAPTER 8

1 Zeydabadi Nejad S, Ramezani Tehrani F, Zadeh-Vakili A. The role of kisspeptin in female reproduction. *Int J Endocrinol Metab*. 2017 Apr 22;15(3):e44337. doi:10.5812/ijem.44337.

2 Schmidt SL, Bessesen DH, Stotz S, et al. Adrenergic control of lipolysis in women compared with men. *J Appl Physiol* (1985). 2014;117(9):1008–19. doi:10.1152/japplphysiol.00003.2014.

3 Dirlewanger M, di Vetta V, Guenat E, et al. Effects of short-term carbohydrate or fat overfeeding on energy expenditure and plasma leptin concentrations in healthy female subjects. *Int J Obes Relat Metab Disord*. 2000;24(11):1413–18. doi:10.1038/sj.ijo.0801395.

4 Poehlman ET, Tremblay A, Fontaine E, et al. Genotype dependency of the thermic effect of a meal and associated hormonal changes following short-term overfeeding. *Metabolism*. 1986;35(1):30–36. doi:10.1016/0026-0495(86)90092-2.

5 Ivy JL. Glycogen resynthesis after exercise: effect of carbohydrate intake. *Int J Sports Med*. 1998;19 Suppl 2:S142–S145. doi:10.1055/s-2007-971981.

CHAPTER 9

1 Mendes E. Regular soda popular with young, nonwhite, low-income. Gallup. https://news.gallup.com/poll/163997/regular-soda-popular-young-nonwhite-low-income.aspx?ref=image. Published August 15, 2013. Accessed September 4, 2020.

2 Sachmechi I, Khalid A, Awan SI, et al. Autoimmune thyroiditis with hypothyroidism induced by sugar substitutes. *Cureus*. 2018 Sep 7;10(9):e3268. doi:10.7759/cureus.3268.

3 Qin X. Etiology of inflammatory bowel disease: a unified hypothesis. *World J Gastroenterol*. 2012;18(15):1708–22. doi:10.3748/wjg.v18.i15.1708.

4 Abou-Donia MB, El-Masry EM, Abdel-Rahman AA, et al. Splenda alters gut microflora and increases intestinal p-glycoprotein and cytochrome p-450 in male rats. *J Toxicol Environ Health A*. 2008;71(21):1415–29. doi:10.1080/15287390802328630.

5 Farrell RJ, Kelly CP. Celiac sprue. *N Engl J Med*. 2002;346(3):180–88. doi:10.1056/NEJMra010852.

6 Foster-Powell K, Holt SH, Brand-Miller JC. International table of glycemic index and glycemic load values: 2002. *Am J Clin Nutr*. 2002;76(1):5–56. doi:10.1093/ajcn/76.1.5.

7 Schatz IJ, Masaki K, Yano K, et al. Cholesterol and all-cause mortality in elderly people from the Honolulu Heart Program: a cohort study. *Lancet*. 2001;358(9279):351–355. doi:10.1016/S0140-6736(01)05553-2.

8 de Souza RJ, Mente A, Maroleanu A, et al. Intake of saturated and trans unsaturated fatty acids and risk of all cause mortality, cardiovascular disease, and type 2 diabetes: systematic review and meta-analysis of observational studies. *BMJ*. 2015 Aug 11;351:h3978. doi:10.1136/bmj.h3978.

9 Veum VL, Laupsa-Borge J, Eng Ø, et al. Visceral adiposity and metabolic syndrome after very high-fat and low-fat isocaloric diets: a randomized controlled trial. *Am J Clin Nutr*. 2017;105(1):85–99. doi:10.3945/ajcn.115.123463.

10 Reference GH. Lactose intolerance. Genetics Home Reference. https://ghr.nlm.nih.gov/condition/lactose-intolerance#statistics. Accessed September 4, 2020.

11 Alcohol use disorder–Symptoms and causes. Mayo Clinic. Published July 11, 2018. Accessed October 7, 2020. https://www.mayoclinic.org/diseases-conditions/alcohol-use-disorder/symptoms-causes/syc-20369243.

12 American Institute for Cancer Research. https://www.aicr.org/news/new-report-just-one-alcoholic-drink-a-day-increases-breast-cancer-risk-exercise-lowers-risk/. Accessed September 4, 2020.

13 Topiwala A, Allan CL, Valkanova V, et al. Moderate alcohol consumption as risk factor for adverse brain outcomes and cognitive decline: longitudinal cohort study. *BMJ*. 2017 Jun 6;357:j2353. doi:10.1136/bmj.j2353.

14 de Visser RO, Robinson E, Bond R. Voluntary temporary abstinence from alcohol during "Dry January" and subsequent alcohol use. *Health Psychol.* 2016;35(3):281–89. doi:10.1037/hea0000297.

15 Stice E, Davis K, Miller NP, Marti CN. Fasting increases risk for onset of binge eating and bulimic pathology: a 5-year prospective study. *J Abnorm Psychol.* 2008;117(4):941–46. doi:10.1037/a0013644.

16 da Luz FQ, Hay P, Gibson AA, et al. Does severe dietary energy restriction increase binge eating in overweight or obese individuals? A systematic review. *Obes Rev.* 2015;16(8):652–65. doi:10.1111/obr.12295.

CHAPTER 10

1 Press Release: Updated tap water databases and drinking water quality analysis. EWG. https://www.ewg.org/news/news-releases/2009/12/09/press-release-updated-tap-water-databases-and-drinking-water-quality. Accessed September 4, 2020.

2 Duhigg C. Millions drink tap water that is legal, but maybe not healthy. *NYTimes.* https://www.nytimes.com/2009/12/17/us/17water.html. Published December 17, 2009. Accessed September 4, 2020.

3 U.S. Department of Health and Human Services Federal Panel on Community Water Fluoridation. U.S. Public Health Service recommendation for fluoride concentration in drinking water for the prevention of dental caries. *Public Health Rep.* 2015;130(4):318–31. doi:10.1177/003335491513000408.

4 Rebello CJ, Keller JN, Liu AG, et al. Pilot feasibility and safety study examining the effect of medium chain triglyceride supplementation in subjects with mild cognitive impairment: a randomized controlled trial.

BBA Clin. 2015 Jan 16;3:123–25. doi:10.1016/j.bbacli.2015.01.001.

5 Sharma A, Bemis M, Desilets AR. Role of medium chain triglycerides (Axona®) in the treatment of mild to moderate Alzheimer's disease. *Am J Alzheimer's Dis Other Demen.* 2014;29(5):409–14. doi:10.1177/1533317513518650.

6 Rebello CJ, Keller JN, Liu AG, et al. Pilot feasibility and safety study examining the effect of medium chain triglyceride supplementation in subjects with mild cognitive impairment: a randomized controlled trial. *BBA Clin.* 2015 Jan 16;3:123–25. doi:10.1016/j.bbacli.2015.01.001.

7 Fernando WM, Martins IJ, Goozee KG, et al. The role of dietary coconut for the prevention and treatment of Alzheimer's disease: potential mechanisms of action. *Br J Nutr.* 2015;114(1):1–14.

8 Liu YM, Wang HS. Medium-chain triglyceride ketogenic diet, an effective treatment for drug-resistant epilepsy and a comparison with other ketogenic diets. *Biomed J.* 2013;36(1):9–15. doi:10.4103/2319-4170.107154.

9 Shilling M, Matt L, Rubin E, et al. Antimicrobial effects of virgin coconut oil and its medium-chain fatty acids on *Clostridium difficile. J Med Food.* 2013;16(12):1079–85. doi:10.1089/jmf.2012.0303.

10 Kabara JJ, Swieczkowski DM, Conley AJ, Truant JP. Fatty acids and derivatives as antimicrobial agents. *Antimicrob Agents Chemother.* 1972;2(1):23–28. doi:10.1128/aac.2.1.23.

11 St-Onge MP, Mayrsohn B, O'Keeffe M, et al. Impact of medium and long chain triglycerides consumption on appetite and food intake in overweight men. *Eur J Clin Nutr.* 2014;68(10):1134–40. doi:10.1038/ejcn.2014.145.

12 Rial SA, Karelis AD, Bergeron KF, Mounier C. Gut microbiota and metabolic health: the potential beneficial effects of a medium chain triglyceride diet in obese individuals. *Nutrients.* 2016;8(5):281. Published 2016 May 12. doi:10.3390/nu8050281.

13 Nosaka N, Suzuki Y, Nagatoishi A, Kasai M, et al. Effect of ingestion of medium-chain triacylglycerols on moderate- and high-intensity exercise in recreational athletes. *J Nutr Sci Vitaminol* (Tokyo). 2009;55(2):120–25. doi:10.3177/jnsv.55.120.

14 Kondreddy VK, Anikisetty M, Naidu KA. Medium-chain triglycerides and monounsaturated fatty acids potentiate the beneficial effects of fish oil on selected cardiovascular risk factors in rats. *J Nutr Biochem.* 2016;28:91–102. doi:10.1016/j.jnutbio.2015.10.005.

15 Eckel RH, Hanson AS, Chen AY, et al. Dietary substitution of medium-chain triglycerides improves insulin-mediated glucose metabolism in NIDDM subjects. *Diabetes.* 1992;41(5):641–47.

16 Ronis MJ, Korourian S, Zipperman M, et al. Dietary saturated fat reduces alcoholic hepatotoxicity in rats by altering fatty acid metabolism and membrane composition. *J Nutr.* 2004;134(4):904–912. doi:10.1093/jn/134.4.904.

17 Serafini M, Del Rio D, Yao DN, et al. Health benefits of tea. In: Benzie IFF, Wachtel-Galor S, editors. *Herbal Medicine: Biomolecular and Clinical Aspects.* 2nd ed. Boca Raton (FL): CRC Press/Taylor & Francis; 2011. Chapter 12. Available from: https://www.ncbi.nlm.nih.gov/books/NBK92768/.

18 Thring TS, Hili P, Naughton DP. Antioxidant and potential anti-inflammatory activity of extracts and formulations of white tea, rose, and witch hazel on primary human dermal fibroblast cells. *J Inflamm*

(Lond). 2011 Oct 13;8(1):27. doi:10.1186/1476-9255-8-27.

19 Wolfram S. Effects of green tea and EGCG on cardiovascular and metabolic health. *J Am Coll Nutr.* 2007;26(4):373S–388S. doi:10.1080/07315724.2007.10719626.

20 Weiss DJ, Anderton CR. Determination of catechins in matcha green tea by micellar electrokinetic chromatography. *J Chromatogr A.* 2003;1011(1-2):173–80. doi:10.1016/s0021-9673(03)01133-6.

21 He RR, Chen L, Lin BH, et al. Beneficial effects of oolong tea consumption on diet-induced overweight and obese subjects. *Chin J Integr Med.* 2009;15(1):34–41. doi:10.1007/s11655-009-0034-8.

22 Yang Y, Qiao L, Zhang X, et al. Effect of methylated tea catechins from Chinese oolong tea on the proliferation and differentiation of 3T3-L1 preadipocyte. *Fitoterapia.* 2015;104:45–49. doi:10.1016/j.fitote.2015.05.007.

23 Leung LK, Su Y, Chen R, et al. Theaflavins in black tea and catechins in green tea are equally effective antioxidants. *J Nutr.* 2001;131(9):2248–51. doi:10.1093/jn/131.9.2248.

24 Russo R, Cassiano MG, Ciociaro A, et al. Role of D-Limonene in autophagy induced by bergamot essential oil in SH-SY5Y neuroblastoma cells. *PLoS One.* 2014 Nov 24;9(11):e113682. doi:10.1371/journal.pone.0113682.

25 Han WY, Zhao FJ, Shi YZ, et al. Scale and causes of lead contamination in Chinese tea. *Environ Pollut.* 2006;139(1):125–132. doi:10.1016/j.envpol.2005.04.025.

26 Amsterdam JD, Shults J, Soeller I, et al. Chamomile (*Matricaria recutita*) may provide antidepressant activity in anxious, depressed humans: an exploratory study. *Altern Ther Health Med.* 2012;18(5):44–49.

27 Sarris J, Stough C, Bousman CA, et al. Kava in the treatment of generalized anxiety disorder: a double-blind, randomized, placebo-controlled study. *J Clin Psychopharmacol.* 2013;33(5):643–48. doi:10.1097/JCP.0b013e318291be67.

28 Akhondzadeh S, Naghavi HR, Vazirian M, et al. Passionflower in the treatment of generalized anxiety: a pilot double-blind randomized controlled trial with oxazepam. *J Clin Pharm Ther.* 2001;26(5):363–67. doi:10.1046/j.1365-2710.2001.00367.

29 Chu W, Cheung SCM, Lau RAW, et al. Bilberry (*Vaccinium myrtillus* L.) In: Benzie IFF, Wachtel-Galor S, editors. *Herbal Medicine: Biomolecular and Clinical Aspects.* 2nd ed. Boca Raton (FL): CRC Press/Taylor & Francis; 2011. Chapter 4. Available from: https://www.ncbi.nlm.nih.gov/books/NBK92770/.

30 Preuss HG, Echard B, Bagchi D, Stohs S. Inhibition by natural dietary substances of gastrointestinal absorption of starch and sucrose in rats and pigs: 1. Acute studies. *Int J Med Sci.* 2007 Aug 6;4(4):196–202. doi:10.7150/ijms.4.196.

31 Al-Dujaili EA, Kenyon CJ, Nicol MR, Mason JI. Liquorice and glycyrrhetinic acid increase DHEA and deoxycorticosterone levels in vivo and in vitro by inhibiting adrenal SULT2A1 activity. *Mol Cell Endocrinol.* 2011;336(1-2):102–9. doi:10.1016/j.mce.2010.12.011.

32 Schloms L, Smith C, Storbeck KH, et al. Rooibos influences glucocorticoid levels and steroid ratios in vivo and in vitro: a natural approach in the management of stress and metabolic disorders? *Mol Nutr Food Res.* 2014;58(3):537–49. doi:10.1002/mnfr.201300463.

33 Harrington AM, Hughes PA, Martin CM, et al. A novel role for TRPM8 in visceral afferent function. *Pain.*

2011;152(7):1459–68. doi:10.1016/j.pain.2011.01.027.

34 Krawitz C, Mraheil MA, Stein M, et al. Inhibitory activity of a standardized elderberry liquid extract against clinically-relevant human respiratory bacterial pathogens and influenza A and B viruses. *BMC Complement Altern Med.* 2011 Feb 25;11:16. doi:10.1186/1472-6882-11-16.

35 Johnson TA, Sohn J, Inman WD, et al. Lipophilic stinging nettle extracts possess potent anti-inflammatory activity, are not cytotoxic and may be superior to traditional tinctures for treating inflammatory disorders. *Phytomedicine.* 2013;20(2):143–47. doi:10.1016/j.phymed.2012.09.016.

36 Mashhadi NS, Ghiasvand R, Askari G, et al. Anti-oxidative and anti-inflammatory effects of ginger in health and physical activity: review of current evidence. *Int J Prev Med.* 2013;4(Suppl 1):S36–S42.

37 Cohen M. Rosehip–an evidence based herbal medicine for inflammation and arthritis. *Aust Fam Physician.* 2012;41(7):495–98.

38 Reinagel NDM. Getting more sleep can reduce food cravings. *Scientific American.* https://www.scientificamerican.com/article/getting-more-sleep-can-reduce-food-cravings/. Published October 22, 2019. Accessed September 4, 2020.

39 Henst RHP, Pienaar PR, Roden LC, Rae DE. The effects of sleep extension on cardiometabolic risk factors: a systematic review. *J Sleep Res.* 2019;28(6):e12865. doi:10.1111/jsr.12865.

40 VanHelder T, Symons JD, Radomski MW. Effects of sleep deprivation and exercise on glucose tolerance. *Aviat Space Environ Med.* 1993;64(6):487–92.

41 Spiegel K, Leproult R, Van Cauter E. Impact of sleep debt on metabolic and endocrine function. *Lancet.*

1999;354(9188):1435–39. doi:10.1016/S0140-6736(99)01376-8.

42 Kato M, Phillips BG, Sigurdsson G, et al. Effects of sleep deprivation on neural circulatory control. *Hypertension.* 2000;35(5):1173–75. doi:10.1161/01.hyp.35.5.1173.

43 Shearer WT, Reuben JM, Mullington JM, et al. Soluble TNF-alpha receptor 1 and IL-6 plasma levels in humans subjected to the sleep deprivation model of spaceflight. *J Allergy Clin Immunol.* 2001;107(1):165–70. doi:10.1067/mai.2001.112270.

44 Meier-Ewert HK, Ridker PM, Rifai N, et al. Effect of sleep loss on C-reactive protein, an inflammatory marker of cardiovascular risk. *J Am Coll Cardiol.* 2004;43(4):678–83. doi:10.1016/j.jacc.2003.07.050.

45 Lack of sleep is affecting Americans, finds the National Sleep Foundation | Sleep Foundation. Sleep Foundation. https://www.sleepfoundation.org/press-release/lack-sleep-affecting-americans-finds-national-sleep-foundation. Accessed September 4, 2020.

46 Reports BCCR. Why Americans can't sleep. *Consumer Reports.* https://www.consumerreports.org/sleep/why-americans-cant-sleep/. Accessed September 4, 2020.

47 Sullivan Bisson AN, Robinson SA, Lachman ME. Walk to a better night of sleep: testing the relationship between physical activity and sleep. *Sleep Health.* 2019;5(5):487–94. doi:10.1016/j.sleh.2019.06.003.

48 Zick SM, Wright BD, Sen A, Arnedt JT. Preliminary examination of the efficacy and safety of a standardized chamomile extract for chronic primary insomnia: a randomized placebo-controlled pilot study. *BMC Complement Altern Med.* 2011 Sep 22;11:78. doi:10.1186/1472-6882-11-78.

49 Abbasi B, Kimiagar M, Sadeghniiat K, et al. The effect of magnesium supplementation on primary insomnia in elderly: A double-blind placebo-controlled clinical trial. *J Res Med Sci.* 2012;17(12):1161–69.

50 Feeney KA, Hansen LL, Putker M, et al. Daily magnesium fluxes regulate cellular timekeeping and energy balance. *Nature.* 2016;532(7599):375–79. doi:10.1038/nature17407.

51 Office of Dietary Supplements–Valerian. https://ods.od.nih.gov/factsheets/Valerian-HealthProfessional/. Accessed September 4, 2020.

52 Ota M, Wakabayashi C, Sato N, et al. Effect of L-theanine on glutamatergic function in patients with schizophrenia. *Acta Neuropsychiatr.* 2015;27(5):291–96. doi:10.1017/neu.2015.22.

53 Lyon MR, Kapoor MP, Juneja LR. The effects of L-theanine (Suntheanine®) on objective sleep quality in boys with attention deficit hyperactivity disorder (ADHD): a randomized, double-blind, placebo-controlled clinical trial. *Altern Med Rev.* 2011;16(4):348–54.

54 Herxheimer A, Petrie KJ. Melatonin for the prevention and treatment of jet lag. *Cochrane Database Syst Rev.* 2002;(2):CD001520. doi:10.1002/14651858.CD001520.

55 Aird TP, Davies RW, Carson BP. Effects of fasted vs fed-state exercise on performance and post-exercise metabolism: a systematic review and meta-analysis. *Scand J Med Sci Sports.* 2018;28(5):1476–93. doi:10.1111/sms.13054.

56 Van Proeyen K, Szlufcik K, Nielens H, et al. Training in the fasted state improves glucose tolerance during fat-rich diet. *J Physiol.* 2010;588(Pt 21):4289–4302. doi:10.1113/jphysiol.2010.196493.

57 Melanson EL, MacLean PS, Hill JO. Exercise improves fat metabolism in muscle but does not increase 24-h fat oxidation. *Exerc Sport Sci Rev.* 2009;37(2):93–101. doi:10.1097/JES.0b013e31819c2f0b.

58 Publishing HH. Walking: your steps to health–Harvard Health. Harvard Health. https://www.health.harvard.edu/staying-healthy/walking-your-steps-to-health. Published August 2009. Accessed September 4, 2020.

59 Bassett DR, Schneider PL, Huntington GE. Physical activity in an Old Order Amish community. *Med Sci Sports Exerc.* 2004;36(1):79–85. doi:10.1249/01.MSS.0000106184.71258.32.

60 Garden FL, Jalaludin BB. Impact of urban sprawl on overweight, obesity, and physical activity in Sydney, Australia. *J Urban Health.* 2009;86(1):19–30. doi:10.1007/s11524-008-9332-5.

61 van den Berg MM, Maas J, Muller R, et al. Autonomic nervous system responses to viewing green and built settings: differentiating between sympathetic and parasympathetic activity. *Int J Environ Res Public Health.* 2015 Dec 14;12(12):15860–74. doi:10.3390/ijerph121215026.

62 Parks and improved mental health and quality of life | Fact Sheets | Parks and Health | National Recreation and Park Association. https://www.nrpa.org/our-work/Three-Pillars/health-wellness/ParksandHealth/fact-sheets/parks-improved-mental-health-quality-life/#:~:text=People%20living%20more%20than%201,meters%20from%20a%20green%20space.&text=Results%20also%20showed%20that%20the,the%20less%20stress%20they%20experienced. Accessed September 4, 2020.

Index

About the Author

DR. WILL COLE, IFMCP, DNM, DC, is a leading functional medicine expert who consults with people around the world via webcam at www.drwillcole.com and locally in Pittsburgh, Pennsylvania. Named one of the top fifty functional-medicine and integrative doctors in the nation, Dr. Cole specializes in clinically investigating underlying factors of chronic disease and customizing a functional medicine approach for thyroid issues, auto-immune conditions, hormonal imbalances, digestive disorder, and brain problems. He is the bestselling author of *Ketotarian* and *The Inflammation Spectrum*. Dr. Cole also hosts the popular podcasts *goopfellas* and *The Art of Being Well*. You can find him on Instagram at Instagram.com/drwillcole or on Facebook at facebook.com/doctorwillcole.